YOGA MALA

YOGA MALA

SRI K. PATTABHI JOIS

NORTH POINT PRESS

A DIVISION OF FARRAR, STRAUS AND GIROUX

NEW YORK

North Point Press
A division of Farrar, Straus and Giroux
18 West 18th Street, New York 10011

Distributed in Canada by D&M Publishers, Inc.
Printed in the United States of America
Originally published in the Kannada language in 1962 in India by Sri K. Pattabhi Jois
First English language edition published in 1999 in the United States by
Eddie Stern/Patanjali Yoga Shala
Published in 2002 by North Point Press
This edition, 2010

Archival photographs of Sri K. Pattabhi Jois courtesy of Sri K. Pattabhi Jois
Photographs of Sharath Rangaswamy copyright © 1999 by Stephan Crasneanscki

Library of Congress Control Number: 2002104086
ISBN: 978-0-86547-751-3

www.fsgbooks.com

21   20   19

With reverence

I dedicate the first edition of *Yoga Mala*

at the feet of my esteemed Guru

Mimamsa Tirtha Vedanta Vagisha

Sankhya Yoga Shikarmani

Sri Tirumali Krishnamacharya

WE HAVE SEEN THE TEXT OF YOGA MALA WRITTEN BY MR. K. PATTABHI JOIS. After a deep study of the philosophy and practice of yoga and a personal enjoyment of its fruits, he is now endeavoring to spread its knowledge and benefits. As a result of his extensive knowledge and his in-depth study of yoga philosophy and practices, he is keenly aware of its many intricacies. The text of *Yoga Mala* is the fruit of his labor.

Many people are under the impression that yoga is fit only for those who are free from passions and attachment. While it is true that some aspects of yoga are pertinent to ascetics alone, many others have common application. Various postures, breathing techniques, and other restraints and self controls contribute not only to physical health, but to mental health as well.

A knowledge of these various restraints and controls is necessary to the practice of yoga. In addition, some illnesses considered incurable by modern medicine may be curable by yogic postures and breath control. Which posture is suited to which illness is very well described in *Yoga Mala*.

I hope this primer, compiled by the yoga expert Mr. K. Pattabhi Jois, will be published and will prove beneficial to a great many people.

I RECOMMEND THIS LITTLE BOOK, WHICH IS AN INTRODUCTION TO THE elements of yoga. Vidvan Pattabhi Jois has explained in simple language the philosphy and discipline of *ashtanga* yoga, based on authentic Sanskrit texts. Yoga is India's greatest contribution to humanity. Yoga is an ethic, discipline, and path of spiritual life. Its aim is the purification of the mind and body. It is a perfect way of life. It is necessary nowadays to expound in our regional languages the wisdom contained in Sanskrit texts, as Sanskrit language is not as popular as it once was. We can never lose the treasures of our culture, and it is a duty enjoined on all those who have access to the original sources of our ancient culture to communicate it for the benefit of others. I welcome this book as a right effort made in that direction, and I hope also that Vidvan Pattabhi Jois will continue to write books on other aspects of our culture and philosophy.

Prof. N. A. Nikam, M.A.
Vice-Chancellor, University of Mysore
9th February 1962

THIS TEXT CONCERNING THE SCIENCE OF YOGA AND ITS THERAPEUTIC VALUE IS well-timed. There is a new awakening of interest in yoga in India and other countries thanks to articles in newspapers, as well as other writings.

Knowledge about this philosophy at present is available only in Sanskrit and in a few English texts. Texts, however, in the Kannada language are rare. The author of *Yoga Mala* has admirably filled this void. In addition to his spiritual knowledge and insights into yoga, Mr. K. Pattabhi Jois has practical experience in the subject, which adds luster to his work. I thank the author for his service.

I hope all readers will take advantage of this book. Needless to say, it is a must for students of *Ayurveda*. In addition, modern physicians specializing in the treatment of mental illness will undoubtedly find it useful.

M. Yamunacharya, M.A.
Formerly of the Department of Philosophy
University of Mysore, 1962

CONTENTS

TABLE OF FIGURES

Foreword

Pattbahi Jois (Guruji) was a legend in the practice of yoga. I studied with him for twenty years, and was continuously amazed at how great he was in his personal practice. The parampara of Rama Mohan Brahmachari and Sri T. Krishnamacharya carried on with Guruji, who spent decades under the tutelage of Krishnamacharya, poring over yoga texts and, more important, practicing every facet of yoga with the intent of profoundly understanding its philosophical implications. One can only become a yogi and a great guru after having experienced yoga fully, as my grandfather did.

Fully dedicated to yoga from the time he arrived in Mysore at age twelve, Guruji led a disciplined yet simple life. Deeply devoted to his practices, he would rise early each morning to perform chanting and prayers and, when he was younger, his *asana* practice as well. Above all, he was committed to passing on his knowledge to his students with a passion we all admired, teaching tirelessly at his yoga institute for seventy years. "Yoga is ninety-nine percent practice and one percent theory" is an idea that Guruji repeatedly presented. He meant that we cannot be mechanical in our approach or resort to being only philosophical about yoga; we must engage it practically in our daily life, and gain an understanding of each of the eight limbs. Beyond *asanas*, there are the observances of *yama* and *niyama*—how we conduct ourselves with the world in a kind and aware manner, and how we abide by our own code of morality. By following these observances, one becomes a good yogi.

The book that Guruji used to convey these teachings, *Yoga Mala*, refers to many authoritative yoga texts to support his teachings: Patanjali's *Yoga Sutras*, *Hatha Yoga Pradipika*, many of the Yoga Upanisads, as well the *Yoga Korunta*, a rare text that to this day has only been spoken of by his guru, Krishnamacharya. It took Guruji three years to write *Yoga Mala*, after painstaking research in each authoritative text and manuscript to ensure that his information was credible and not based on fancy. The unique aspect of Krishnamacharya's teaching was *vinyasa karma*, the systematic method of linking breath and movement, and *Yoga Mola* covers this topic in depth.

Guruji instructed countless thousands of people around the world, and guided many to become teachers as well. The method explained in this book is identical to the method taught at his institute in Mysore, the method we follow today. It was his hope that future generations will continue to do the same, and practice in order to preserve the traditional yogic knowledge.

Guruji created a strong foundation of yoga for us by teaching with such dedication for so many years. It is our duty to build upon that foundation so that, in this modern and confusing age, yoga can be passed on undiluted and in its purest form. Guruji dedicated ninety-three years to teaching, and from him we should learn, be inspired, and carry on.

—R. Sharath
Mysore
October 12, 2009

Foreword

SRI KRISHNA PATTABHI JOIS (1915–2009) WAS BORN ON THE FULL MOON DAY of July in the small village of Kowshika, in a district of Hassan, in Karnataka State, South India. Kowshika remains largely unchanged since Guruji spent the first thirteen years of his life there. Then, as now, its three old temples were fixtures in the daily lives of sixty to seventy hardworking village families. Kowshika began to receive electricity only in the 1980s; in Guruji's youth a man with a bicycle was considered rich.

Guruji's father was an astrologer, priest, and landholder. His mother took care of the house and the nine children—five girls and four boys— of whom Jois was the fifth. From the age of five he was instructed in Sanskrit and rituals by his father, as were all Brahmin boys. Later he began studies at the middle school in Hassan, four or five kilometers from Kowshika. No one else in his family had learned yoga or even professed interest in it. In those days in India, yoga was considered an esoteric practice suitable for monks, *sadhus*, and *sannyasis* but not for the householder, who might lose all worldly interest and abandon his family by undertaking the practice.

In the secret text of the yogis, the *Bhagavad Gita*, Krishna proclaims that one comes to yoga in his life only by having practiced it in a previous life, and is pulled toward it against one's will, as toward a magnet—a verse that Guruji was very fond of quoting. It is this type of pull that must have led Guruji to attend a lecture-demonstration a friend told him was being given at the Jubilee Hall of Hassan's middle school in the Indian month of October–November 1927. Jois was amazed by the *asanas*, and by the strong, graceful yogi jumping from pose to pose. Although he didn't understand the lecture, and it was quite some time before he understood the method and philosophy, he liked the yoga and decided to learn it himself. The next day he rose early and went to the house where the yogi was staying. Bravely for a boy of only twelve, he requested to be instructed in yoga. The yogi gruffly demanded of him, Who are you? What is your name? Who is your father? What does he do? Jois dutifully replied, and was told to come back the next day. He began what was to be a twenty-five-year period of study with the great yogi Sri T. Krishnamacharya.

For two years Jois remained in Kowshika and practiced with Krishnamacharya every day. He was young, his body was flexible, and he quickly learned all of the *asanas*. Krishnamacharya was pleased, and used him to perform demonstrations. Jois never told his family he was practicing yoga. He would rise early, go to practice, and then go to school. In 1930, Jois's father performed his Brahmin thread ceremony—the initiation through which all Brahmin boys pass into adulthood and into their spiritual life. Around this time, Krishnamacharya also left Kowshika, to continue spreading his teachings of yoga. Soon afterward, without informing anyone, Guruji left Kowshika for Mysore, with two rupees in his pocket, to attend the maharaja's Sanskrit College. For one or two years he begged for food and slept in the dormitory room of a friend. It was three years before he wrote to tell his father where he was. Jois remained at the College from 1930 to 1956, studying Sanskrit and then the *Vedas*, and eventually earning a professorship in Advaita Vedanta. He taught there until 1973, when he left to devote himself fully to teaching yoga at his yoga *shala*.

His reunion with Krishnamacharya and the beginning of his association with the Maharaja of Mysore took place in 1931. Without knowing who the visiting yogi was, Jois attended a yoga demonstration at the Sanskrit College. To his surprise, he discovered it was his own guru, Krishnamacharya. He was very happy, and prostrated himself at the feet of his teacher. Also present at the demonstration was a minister from the Maharaja of Mysore's palace. The maharaja, Krishna Rajendra Wodeyar, who had a great affinity for yoga and spirituality, was ill. When he heard through his minister about the visiting yogi, he sent for him. Krishnamacharya, with his vast knowledge and healing abilities, was able to cure the maharaja where others had failed. The maharaja became Krishnamacharya's patron, and established a yoga *shala* for him on the palace grounds. Krishnamacharya was to remain in Mysore for the next twenty-two years.

The maharaja became a great patron of yoga, sending Krishnamacharya, along with Guruji and other students at the yoga *shala*, all over India to perform demonstrations, study texts, and research yoga schools and styles. Guruji says today that after having traveled around India for many years, Krishnamacharya is the only man he ever met who had full knowledge of true yoga methods.

On occasion, the maharaja, who was fond of yoga demonstrations, would summon Guruji and his friend and fellow student, Mahadev Bhatt, to the palace. At 10 p.m., an attendant would come to their room and command a demonstration for the maharaja at four a.m. At three a.m., Guruji and Bhatt would get up and take cold baths before a car would come to collect them. The maharaja would tell them which asanas he wanted to see; he particularly liked *Kukkutasana* and *Bakasana* B. Afterward, the maharaja himself would do some *asanas*, and then send them home by car. He would give them thirty-five, forty, or fifty rupees— in those days quite a large amount of money. He would tell them, "Keep this money, don't tell your Guru." On the maharaja's birthday one year, both Guruji and Bhatt were presented with silk Hanuman kacchas to wear during practice. Guruji still speaks today of what a kind man the maharaja was.

Guruji would occasionally assist Krishnamacharya in class and teach if he was late. One day the maharaja, who would sometimes attend class at the yoga *shala*, saw this. One week later the maharaja asked Jois to teach yoga at the Sanskrit College. Guruji replied that he had come to Mysore only to study. The maharaja offered him a salary, a scholarship to the college, and room and board. Since Guruji was still begging, this was a lucky opportunity. He told the maharaja he first must ask for Krishnamacharya's blessing. On March 1, 1937, Jois began to teach at the Sanskrit College. When asked if he ever received a teaching certificate, he replied yes, and his test was very difficult: Krishnamacharya gave him one sick man and said, "Fix him!"

Guruji has often spoken about a text called the *Yoga Korunta*, an ancient manuscript on *ashtanga* yoga, which had been the basis of the practical lessons on yoga taught to him by Krishnamacharya. Attributed to the sage Vamana, it was one of the many texts taught orally to Krishnamacharya, which he learned by heart during the seven and a half years he spent living with his teacher, Rama Mohan Brahmachari. *Korunta* means "groups," and the text was said to contain lists of many different groupings of *asanas*, as well as highly original teachings on *vinyasa*, *drishti*, *bandhas*, *mudras*, and philosophy. Before Krishnamacharya was sent off into the world to teach, around 1924, he was told that he could find this text in the Calcutta University Library. According to Guruji, who has never seen the text and doubted that it still exists, Krishnamacharya spent some time in Calcutta researching this book, which was badly damaged and had many missing portions. When Guruji began his studies with Krishnamacharya in 1927, it was the methods from the *Yoga Korunta* that he was taught. Although the authenticity of the book would be extremely difficult, if not impossible, to validate today, it is generally accepted that this is the source of *ashtanga* yoga as taught by Pattabhi Jois.

In 1948, in his home in Lakshmipurum, Guruji established the Ashtanga Yoga Research Institute, with the aim of experimenting with the curative aspect of yoga as taught to him by Krishnamacharya and the ancient texts. The house at that time had only two rooms and a kitchen and bath, and it was not until 1964 that he built an extension in back for the yoga hall, and a resting room upstairs.

About this time a Belgian named André van Lysebeth found his way to Jois. Van Lysebeth knew Sanskrit, and spent two months studying the primary and intermediate *asanas*. Among the many books he was to write was one called *Pranayama*, which included a photo of Guruji along with his name and address. It was through van Lysebeth's book that his whereabouts became known in Europe, and thus the Europeans were the first to come from the West specifically to study with Guruji. In 1973, the first Americans came, after Guruji's son Manju demonstrated yoga at Swami Gitananda's ashram in Pondicherry.

Guruji's first trip to the West was by invitation of Marie Helena Bastidos to a yoga conference she was holding in South America in 1974, where he delivered a talk on yoga in Sanskrit, which was translated into several languages. In 1975 he traveled to California with Manju. He has said on many occasions that only twenty or thirty students practiced *ashtanga* yoga in America then, but, "gradually, gradually, in twenty years, it will be fully spreading." Through his many trips to America over a thirty-year period, Guruji's teaching has borne fruit, and his influence here, direct and indirect, is central to the growth and popularity of yoga in America today.

A portion of the record we have of Guruji's knowledge of yoga comes to us in the form of his writings and photographs. His main treatise, this small book, *Yoga Mala*, outlines the timeless nature of *ashtanga* yoga practice. Guruji began work on it in 1958, writing the entire text by hand, little by little, over a two- to three-year period, in the afternoons while his family rested. It was first published in India in 1962 by one of his students, a coffee planter in Coorg. *Mala* is a Sanskrit term that means garland. In India, there are many different kinds of *malas*. There are *japamalas*, made up of sacred beads strung on a thread which are used in prayer for counting and keeping focused on the repetition of a mantra. There are *pushpamalas*, which are garlands of vivid flowers, smelling of jasmine and other scents, that are strung in the form of wreaths and offered in worship to deities in homes and temples. Guruji here offers another kind of *mala*, which is ancient in tradition, as sacred as a prayer, and as fragrant as flowers. His *mala* is a garland of yoga, in which each *vinyasa* is like a sacred bead to be counted and focused on, and each *asana* is like a flower strung on the thread of the breath. Just as a *japamala* adorns the neck and a *pushpamala* adorns the gods, so too does this garland of yoga, when diligently practiced, adorn our entire being with peace, health, radiance, and, ultimately, self-knowledge.

The translators have tried to remain as faithful as possible to the original, both in style and content. Guruji has rewritten small sections, corrected errors, and made additions to his original work. For example, descriptions of the yoga postures known as *Prasarita Padottanasana* (D) and *Janu Shirshasana* (B & C), which did not appear in the original, have been included here. Some portions of the book have also been rewritten for the sake of clarity, and footnotes have been provided to aid understanding. Every change and addition, however, has been reviewed by Guruji, who has provided information for some of the emendations, and dictated others.

Guruji went against the grain of his times by dedicating his life to teaching yoga. Perhaps that is why he never told his family he was doing yoga, and why he left for Mysore without a word. Maybe they would have protested, tried to talk some sense into his head. It is clear for Guruji there was never any question. He taught without hesitation, neither for fame nor money, although these things may have come to him. Pattabhi Jois was a shining example of pure dedication, of what it takes to keep the light of an ancient tradition burning brightly.

—Eddie Stern
New York City
March 10, 2010

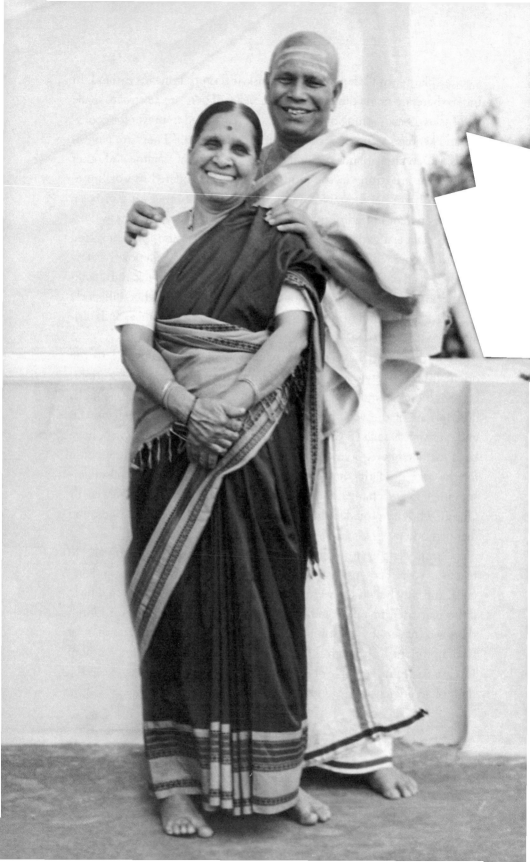

Preface

WHAT A GREAT PLEASURE IT IS THAT YOGIC PRACTICE, WHICH FORMS PART OF our Indian culture, has gained recognition and respect not only in our own country, but in Western countries as well. We know from various scriptures, *puranas*, *Vedas*, and legends that the science of yoga has been in existence in India since time immemorial. We also know that, as years passed and times changed, it reached a very low state. Nonetheless, a knowledge of yoga has always remained very important to all people—men and women.

There are differences of opinion regarding the science of yoga, though in recent times, and to some extent, the situation has altered. There are those, for example, who say that its practice is only a form of physical exercise, with little else to recommend it; according to others, it is useful only to *sannyasins*, or people living an absolute celibate life, and family men should thus abstain from it. Some people even have a fear of practicing it altogether. But this is little different from the opinion of those who look for the faults of sugar without knowing its sweetness. Once they taste it, its sweetness becomes apparent. Similarly, once we practice yoga, we come to realize its *ananda* [bliss].

And yet the practice of yoga still leaves us subject to doubts and misconceptions, which weaken our minds and sense organs. Consequently, we plunge ourselves into the torments of birth and death, and experience various forms of suffering without ever seeing material or spiritual prosperity. Yet we should accept scriptural authority, as the Lord in the *Bhagavad Gita* has ordained: *"Tasmat shastram pramanam te karya akarya vyavasthitau* [Therefore, the sacred teaching (*shastra*) is your measure in determining what is to be done and what is not to be done]." If we practice the science of yoga, which is useful to the entire human community and which yields happiness both here and hereafter—if we practice it without fail, we will then attain physical, mental, and spiritual happiness, and our minds will flood toward the Self. It is with this great desire that I have written this book.

With gratitude,
K. Pattabhi Jois
Mysore, September 1997

YOGA MALA

Sri Gurum Gananatham cha
Vanim shanmathuram tatha
Yogeshwaram Sri Harim cha
Pranat'osmi moohoormuhu.
[To the blessed Guru and Ganesh
As well as to Saraswati and Skanda
To Shiva, the lord of the yogis, and Shri Hari
I bow again and again.]

Source: *Traditional prayer*

Vande Gurunam charanaravinde
Sandarshita svatmasukhavabodhe
Nishreyase jangalikayamane
Samsara halahala mohashantyai.
[I worship the Guru's lotus feet
Awakening the happiness of the Self revealed
Beyond comparison, acting like the jungle physician
To pacify delusion from the poison of existence.]

Source: *Yoga Taravalli* by Shankaracharya

THE PRACTICE OF YOGA IS NOT NEW TO THE PEOPLE OF INDIA. IT IS A NOBLE, desireless action, coupled with righteousness, which has been passed down, in an unbroken tradition, since time immemorial.[1] Many stories are told in our Epics of how the people of India attained divinity by the practice of yoga. Many of our scriptures too speak of how fundamental yoga is, and of how it forms the basis of other sciences. It is thus sad that today, many who call themselves worthy sons of Mother India have not even heard of yoga *vidya* [knowledge]. Once upon a time, people practiced yoga in each and every corner of India. Now, it is the pursuit of pleasure that prevails, and not the pursuit of yoga. People in the world experience yoga, pleasure, or disease, whichever it may be, in accordance with their karma.

---

1 *Nishkama karma* (*nish-* without + *kama* desire : *karma* action) is an action performed without a wish or desire for the "fruits," or results, of such action. The ultimate yogic ideal is to perform all actions without desire for personal gain, and to offer instead the fruits of all actions to God. Performing actions with the mind directed toward results increases ego and keeps us bonded to the idea of "I" and "mine," while offering the fruits of actions to God leads toward surrender to the divine will and liberation from the idea of a separate self.

From pleasure, disease is certain. Some people think that one must be lucky to enjoy pleasure. This, of course, is true. But can it also not be said that, in order to experience disease, one must be lucky as well?

Let us consider the true nature of yoga. We have heard the term used in day-to-day life, as well as in the scriptures, Upanishads, and sutras, and yet it does not seem that we have any precise knowledge of what it means.[2] We know of only one yoga, in the form of asana and pranayama, which is useful to strict brahmacharis [celibates] and sannyasins [renunciates] alone, and not to ordinary men.[3] Yet, if we look into the scriptures properly, understand their meaning, and reflect on them, we will come to know yoga's true nature.

What then is yoga? The word has many meanings: relation; means; union; knowledge; matter; logic; and so on. For now, let us say that the meaning of yoga is upaya, which means path, or way which we follow or by means of which we can attain something. What then is the path we should follow? What or whom should we seek to attain? The mind should seek to attain what is best. Just as a servant seeks a king to serve, a disciple seeks the best Guru, and a wife seeks an ideal husband, so too will the mind seek the Universal Self.[4] Even this is one type of union. As the servant who wins his master's heart and blessings through his virtues and good conduct verily attains royal character himself; and the disciple who, by great virtue and intellectual power, verily wins the heart of his Guru and becomes as one with the Guru; and the wife who shows virtue and character, as well as devotion to her husband, verily becomes as one with her husband, so too, if the mind establishes itself in the Self or attains the Self, it will not exist as different from the Self. Thus, the way of estab-

---

2 The Upanishads form part of the Vedas, or sacred scriptures of Hinduism, and contain the basic doctrines of the faith; the sutras referred to here and throughout the book are generally the Patanjali Yoga Sutras, the authoritative text of ashtanga, or eight-limbed, yoga.

3 Asana, or yogic postures, and pranayama, or breathing exercises, are two of the eight limbs of ashtanga yoga.

4 The phrase "Universal Self" is a translation of the word Atman, the term used by the author in his original manuscript. According to Vedanta, the Atman is the soul of man, and all souls are part of an infinite, all-pervading Supreme Spirit. The term is commonly translated into English as "Supreme Self," "Universal Self," "Indwelling Spirit," or simply "Self," and refers to our higher, unchanging, eternal nature of pure consciousness, truth, and bliss. By contrast, the English word self is used to signify the essential aspects of a person's individuality, including body, mind, and personality, which are all subject to birth, decay, and death, and are therefore not eternal in nature.

lishing the mind in the Self should be known as yoga. An aphorism of Patanjali, the great sage and founder of the science of yoga, makes this clear: "*Yoga chitta vritti nirodhaha* [Yoga is the process of ending the definitions of the field of consciousness]."[5]

It is in the nature of our sense organs to grasp their respective sense objects. If the sense organs are harmonized by the mind, and if the mind establishes itself in the sense organs, then objects are known or grasped. If, however, there is no contact between the mind and the sense organs, knowledge of objects will not occur. The mind is thus the basis of all sensory functions. The means by which the mind is directed toward the Self and prevented from going toward outside objects is what is known as yoga, as a hymn of the *Katha Upanishad* affirms: "*Tham yogam iti manyante sthiram indriya dharanam* [Yoga is considered to be the steady fixing of the senses]."[6] Here, the means to establishing the sense organs in the Indweller, and thus to preventing them from going toward external objects, is called yoga. Therefore, the word *yoga* signifies the means to the realization of one's true nature.

We now have to ask whether it is possible to realize the true nature of yoga simply by understanding its meaning as a word. By the mere study of texts on yoga, by the mere grasp of yoga's meaning as a word, by a mere discussion of the pros and cons of this intellectual grasp, one cannot have a thorough knowledge of yoga. For, just as a good knowledge of culinary science does not satisfy hunger, neither will the benefits of yoga be realized fully by a mere understanding of the science of its practice. Thus, the scriptures only show us the right path. It is left to us to understand them and to put them into practice. By the strength gained through this practice, we can come to know the method for bringing the mind and sense organs under control. Thus can we achieve yoga. For it is only through the control of the mind and sense organs that we come to know our true nature, and not through intellectual knowledge, or by putting on the garb of a yogi.

Hence an aspirant, by the grace of his Guru and constant practice of yoga, can someday realize, before casting off his mortal coil, the Indweller that is of the nature of supreme peace and eternal bliss, and the cause of

---

5 *Patanjali Yoga Sutras* i : 2

6 *Katha Upanishad* ii : 3 : 11

the creation, sustenance, and destruction of the universe. Otherwise, an aspirant will be unable to see anything in this world but turmoil.

HOW CAN WE MAKE THE MIND ONE-POINTED SO THAT WE MAY SEE THE Universal Self? This is what *ashtanga* yoga teaches. The word *ashtanga* means eight limbs, or steps, and these comprise: *yama*; *niyama*; *asana*; *pranayama*; *pratyahara*; *dharana*; *dhyana*; and *samadhi*.

YAMA

Yama, the first limb, consists of five parts: *ahimsa*; *satya*; *asteya*; *brahmacharya*; and *aparigraha*.

AHIMSA

Ahimsa means not causing injury to anyone, including animals, in any form, at any time, or for any reason, in word, thought, or deed. If an injury has Vedic sanction, it does not constitute *ahimsa*. Two animals hostile to each other will forget their hostility in the vicinity of those who practice absolute *ahimsa*.

> *Ahimsa pratishthayam tat sannidhou vairatyagah.*
> [Upon being established in non-hurtfulness, there is
> a relinquishing of hostility in the presence of that (*ahimsa*).]
> — *Patanjali Yoga Sutras* ii : 35

SATYA

What is *satya*? *Satya* is truthfulness. One should always tell the truth in thought, word, and deed. The truth must be pleasant to others; an unpleasant truth should not be uttered. If one follows the truth in this manner, all one's words will become true and all one's desires will be fulfilled.

> *Satya pratishthayam kriya phala shrayatvam.*
> [Upon being established in truth, there is surety in the result of actions.]
> — *Patanjali Yoga Sutras* ii : 36

Asteya means not stealing the property or possessions of others. Being envious of or begrudging another; cheating someone with sweet words; gaining selfish ends under the guise of truthfulness: all are to be abandoned. Heaps of gems fall before the yogi who practices *asteya*, and he becomes the abode of all gems.

> *Asteya pratishthayam sarvaratna upasthanam.*
> [Upon being established in non-stealing, there occurs the
> attainment of all prosperity.]
> — *Patanjali Yoga Sutras* ii : 37

BRAHMACHARYA

Now, let us discuss *brahmacharya*. What is its meaning? Is it merely the retaining of vital fluid?[7] Does it signify unmarried student life? *Brahmacharya* is not possible by means of the mere retention of vital fluid. Becoming one with the supreme Brahman alone is *brahmacharya*. Were the holding of vital fluid itself *brahmacharya*, it would be a thing impossible to do. There are currently many obstacles to the easy practice of this limb of yoga, and our *Shrutis* and *Smritis*, too, speak of eight types of obstacles:[8]

> *Smaranam kirtanam kelih*
> *Prekshanam muhyabhashanam*
> *Sankalpah adhyavasayascha*
> *Kriya nishpattireva cha*
> *Etam maithunam ashtangam pravadanti manishinah.*
> [Remembering; celebrating; amorous play;
> viewing; infatuated discussion; planning;
> determination; and the effort of one who has no partner:
> the wise declare these to be the eight limbs of romantic activity.]

Maintaining *brahmacharya* nowadays is difficult because there are so many things that attract the mind in different directions, such as theaters,

---

7 The vital fluid here referred to is the sexual fluids.

8 The *Shrutis*, or *Vedas*, are sacred teachings revealed by the Supreme Being to the ancient *rishis*; the *Smritis* are religious and traditional laws and codes devised by human authors.

pleasure houses, restaurants, and the like. The preservation of *brahmacharya* is thus an uphill task.

Now, a question arises. If we cannot maintain *brahmacharya*, does it not amount to saying that yoga is impossible for us? No, a man can achieve some degree of *brahmacharya*. If he is to achieve it, however, he must avoid the following as much as possible: mixing with vulgar people; going to crowded areas for recreation; reading vulgar books which disturb the mind; going to theaters and restaurants; and conversing secretly with strangers of the opposite sex. If these are avoided, *brahmacharya* can be preserved in part. For it is by *brahmacharya* alone that we are able to achieve impossible tasks: to live longer; to conquer death; and, above all, to know the true Self. This is the substance of Patanjali's *sutra*: "*Brahmacharya pratishtayam virya labhah* [Upon being established in *brahmacharya*, vital energy is obtained]." We should thus first seek to preserve this yogic limb.

As Patanjali's *sutra* clearly states, a gain in vitality is *brahmacharya's* fruit. If a gain in vitality is the fruit and, in the case of householders, there is occasion for a loss of vital fluid, does it mean that a householder cannot attain *brahmacharya*? This, of course, is true: householders lose *brahmacharya* owing to seminal loss. With the loss, they lose the strength of their bodies, minds, and sense organs; in addition, *moksha* [spiritual liberation] and the capacity to perceive the soul or realize the true Self become impossible. In the absence of the knowledge of one's own Self, one remains in the cycle of birth and death, and thus must continue to suffer in this sapless and despicable world. However, understanding properly the meanings of the words *brahmacharya* and *virya labhah*, and then putting them into practice, leads us to the supreme goal.

> *Tasmat shastram pramanam te karyakarya vyavasthitou*
> *Jnatva shastra vidhanoktam karma kartumiharhasi*
> [Therefore, the sacred teaching (*shastra*) is your measure in determining what is to be done and what is not to be done. Knowing what is said in the *shastra*, you should act, here in this world.]
> — Bhagavad Gita xvi : 24

In accordance with these divine words, it is important for us to study the scriptures perfectly, to understand their import properly, and to bring them into practice. The scriptures should never be neglected, for they have been given to us for our upliftment. If we denounce them, and behave like animals instead of following their path, then there will be nothing but ruin in store for us. Hence, the righteous path of the scriptures is vital.

Among the stages of life, the second is that of the householder.[9] If we take only seminal loss into account, then a householder cannot attain *mukti* [spiritual liberation]. However, when we consult the scriptures, we find it said that, for householders, seminal loss by itself does not endanger *brahmacharya* and that, in the truest sense of the word, the householder alone can attain *brahmacharya*. In the words of the mantra:

> *Ye diva ratya samyujyante pranameva praskandante*
> *Tatryrudrarau rathya samyujyante brahmacharyam eva*
> [Those who daily engage their energy through romantic
> activity truly dissipate (their energy). Those who take delight
> when the enemy of Shiva (Kama/Cupid) is in decline indeed
> engage in *brahmacharya*.]

By examining this scriptural statement, we come to know that if a man has sexual intercourse with his wife during the daytime, his power of vitality will be lost and, in a very short time, death will conquer him. To counter this, the young men of today offer a different argument. They say, "If a man has sexual intercourse with his lawful wife during the day, his power of vitality is, of course, decreased. Agreed! But what about sex with other women? Where is the fault in that?!" This is only the question of perverted rationalists. Intercourse with other women is always forbidden and, as has been said before, it is, even mentally, harmful to *brahmacharya*.

Leaving that aside, the *shastrakaras* state that if sexual intercourse is engaged in only at night and in accordance with the menstrual periods, then even householders and the like can be regarded as *brahmacharis*.[10] But

---

9 Indian tradition recognizes four stages (*asramas*) of life. The first is called *brahmacarin*, or the stage of the student; the second is *grhastha*, the householder stage; the third is *vanaprashtha*, or the hermit or anchorite stage; and the fourth, *sannyasin*, is the stage of complete renunciation.

10 The *shastrakaras* are the authors of the *shastras*, which are sacred texts or books of divine authority.

the matter of day and night, as well as of the appropriate time for copulation, have to be taken into consideration. Normally, we consider day as the period from sunrise to sunset. Similarly, we consider night as the period from sunset until the time of the sun's rising again. However, the way of determining day and night for yogis is different. Of the nostrils of the nose through which we breathe, the right one is known as *surya nadi*, and the left one, as *chandra nadi*.[11] For yogis, day and night are determined on the basis of these two *nadis*. During the day, meaning from sunrise to sunset, the two *nadis* are not to be heeded. However, during the nighttime, their transformation should be considered. If, during the night, the breath is felt to be moving through the *surya nadi*, that is, if the wind is coming and going through the right nostril, then that is to be regarded as the daytime and, during that period, copulation and the like are not to occur. If, during the night, on the other hand, the breath is moving only through the *chandra nadi*, then that is the occasion for sexual activities. (Should the *chandra nadi* become active during the daytime, however, it must not be taken as an occasion for engaging in sexual activities.) In this way should householders who are righteous—whether they be yogis or not—ascertain day and night.

In addition to the matter of day and night, the menstrual cycle must also be considered. The interval between the fourth and sixteenth day of a woman's cycle is regarded as the correct time for intercourse by scriptural experts. Beyond the sixteenth day, however, it ceases to be correct; vitality will be lost and the act will not be fruitful following intercourse after the sixteenth day. When we accept the stage of the householder, we make a promise to God, Guru, and our parents in this way. We also make a promise

---

11 A *nadi* [flute-shaped channel] is a tube or hollow nerve pathway. *Nadis* are of three types: the gross, subtle, and very subtle. Called *dhamini*, the first type carries blood, water, and air. The second type is simply termed *nadi*, and it carries energy in the form of *prana* throughout the nervous system. *Sira*, the third, is the smallest and most subtle of all the *nadis*, as small as a human hair that has been split six times. This *nadi* quickly carries messages from the "message center" located in the region of the heart throughout the body, and is also a vital link in the functioning of the sense organs. Any sensory input from the outside world that stimulates the hearing, taste, smell, sight, or touch is communicated to the internal consciousness via the *sira nadi*, which reaches throughout every part of the body. Of the 72,000 *nadis* in the subtle body, three are especially important for yogis: the *surya nadi*; *chandra nadi*; and *sushumna nadi*. The *surya nadi* carries our "sun" energy, or active and hot aspect, and the *chandra nadi* carries our "moon" energy, cooling and tranquil. Our spiritual energy is carried by the pathway of the *sushumna nadi*, which remains closed off until the *surya* and *chandra nadis* have been harmonized through yogic practice.

that we will do nothing apart from our lawful wife with respect to *dharma*, *artha*, and *kama* [righteousness, wealth, and desire, respectively]. Hence it is very important that we beget legal progeny. Engaged in after the sixteenth day, as well as on the days of the new and full moons, the transitory day of the sun (when the sun monthly enters a new constellation), and the eighth and fourteenth days after the full and new moons, sexual intercourse and the like are not related to *brahmacharya*. Union with one's lawful wife should be undertaken for the sake of begetting good progeny, and only after determining the *vitu* [period between the 4th and 16th days] and *kala* [time], and not on any other days, not even in the mind. Thus, in view of the fact that scriptural experts inform us that a householder who follows the injunctions and rules can be regarded as a *brahmacharin*, then even a family man becomes highly eligible for the practice of yoga, due to his ability to preserve his *brahmacharya*. Thus, *brahmacharya* does not mean the holding of vitality, though there is still no room for its squandering.

In truth, establishing the mind in the supreme Brahman, without allowing it to wander here and there, is *brahmacharya*. The word *veerya* means vitality. The transformation of the thirty-second drop of blood is *veerya*, or *dhatu* [semen].[12] If the strength of the mind, as well as of the sense organs, is to be preserved, then the strength of the *dhatu*, which is the effect of the blood's transformation, must also be preserved. If *dhatu* is lost, the strength of the mind, as well as that of the sense organs, will also be lost, and it will not be possible to perceive the nature of the Self. Therefore, to say that from *brahmacharya* there will be a gain in vitality is to say that if the mind turns toward the Inner Self for the sake of knowing the nature of the Self, then the strength will increase. Conversely, if the mind is interested in external objects, then the strength will be dimininished. From the scriptural statement, "*Nayam atma balahinena labhyah* [The Self cannot be gained by the weak]," we see that mental strength is greater

---

12 It is believed that the food we eat is transformed, over a period of thirty-two days, into a single drop of blood. After thirty-two drops of blood have been distilled, thirty-two days must pass for these drops to, in turn, become one drop of vitality. After thirty-two drops of vitality have been generated and, again, thirty-two days have passed, one drop of *amrita bindu*, called the nectar of immortality, is produced. Stored in the head, *bindu* lends strength and shine to the body and mind. When the store of *bindu* decreases, the life span is shortened. But when *bindu* is preserved through *brahmacharya* and the practice of *viparita karani* (*see fn. 44 and Yoga Asanas section*), health, longevity, and mental clarity all increase.

than physical strength. Therefore, if the mind is to be steadied and brought to concentration, it must contemplate the Supreme Self at all times. In other words, whether working, sleeping, eating, playing, or even enjoying intercourse with one's wife—that is, during the three states of experience, namely waking, dreaming, and deep sleep, and in all objects—one should think of the Supreme Self at all times. If the mind is thus given to the constant thought of the Supreme Self, then its strength will increase. And it is this strength that should be regarded as *brahmacharya*.

If *brahmacharya* of this kind is achieved, then the capacity to realize the Self, which is the result of a gain in vitality, will be attained. With this, the *dhatu*, which is the effect of the transformation of the blood, will not be lost, but will continue to nourish the body properly. Only the strong, not the weak, can perceive the Self, as the scriptural statement above tells us. Therefore, the meaning of the phrase *virya labhah* is indeed correct. Hence, the great importance of *brahmacharya*.

> *Brahmacharya pratishthayam virya labhah.*
> [Upon being established in *brahmacharya*, there is the attainment of vital energy.]
> — *Patanjali Yoga Sutras* ii : 38

APARIGRAHA

What is *aparigraha*? If the mortal body is to be sustained, things like food are essential. After all, by sustaining the body, does one not attain divinity through following the righteous path? Thus, the food we eat should be pure (*sattvic*), untainted (*nirmala*), and acquired through righteousness, and not be secured by cheating, deceit, persecution, or other unjust means. Only taking as much food as we need to maintain our bodies, and not desiring things of enjoyment which are superfluous to the physical body, is *aparigraha*. If the limb called *aparigraha* is firmly practiced, details of previous and future births are revealed to the yogi.

> *Aparigraha sthairye janma kathamta sambodhah.*
> [Upon a foundation of non-possessiveness, there arises the full understanding of the wherefore of birth.]
> — *Patanjali Yoga Sutras* ii : 39

EACH OF THE FIVE SUB-LIMBS ABOVE IS ASSOCIATED WITH YAMA, THE FIRST limb, and only the actions of previous lives will lead us to practice them. Thus, the mind will turn itself to the practice of yoga only when a *samskara* or *vasana* is present.[13] Yet even where a *samskara* exists, aspirants must expect to practice the yogic steps with effort.

NIYAMA
We come now to a discussion of *niyama*,
the second step, which has five sub-limbs: *shaucha; santosha;*
tapas; swadhyaya; and *ishwarapranidhana.*

SHAUCHA
There are two types of *shaucha*, or purification: *bahir shaucha* [external purification] and *antah shaucha* [internal purification].

Bahir shaucha, the first, involves washing the outer part of the body with red clay and water. By rubbing the body with clay, sweat and dirt are removed, and the body becomes soft and shiny.

The second, *antah shaucha*, means viewing everything and every being as a friend, and treating all with affection (*maitri*). This means engaging the mind with the supreme feeling that all are our friends, and considering everything to be a reflection of God. Such focusing of our attention on the Supreme Being is *antah shaucha*.

From this twofold *shaucha*, a loathing is developed for the body, which is seen as abominable, essenceless, and perishable, and a disgust is felt when touching the body of another. It is then that one feels the body's purity and thus hesitates to indulge in sin.

---

13 It is believed that only an association with the practice of yoga in a past life will lead to its practice in the present life; to come to yoga, in other words, an inclination, desire, or yearning for it must already exist in one's consciousness. Everything we experience is imprinted upon our conciousness. Each imprint gives rise to an attraction or aversion for the repetition of the experience. Each imprint, or subtle impression, is called *samskara*. The attraction or aversion that arises from it is called *vasana*, which literally means "fragrance." Our entire personality is made up of these countless "fragrances." To deepen this *samskara* in an effort to proceed further along the yogic pattern and path, an aspirant must practice with even greater diligence; otherwise, an impression will not be formed. *Samskara* or *vasana* is likened by Pattabhi Jois to cooking garlic in a pot. If the garlic is boiled for a considerable period of time, then removed and the pot cleaned, its smell will linger on in the pot for a long time. Thus an aspirant who, in a past life, was an American engineer and who, in this life, has been born into a Brahmin family, will find his or her mind drawn toward engineering.

Shauchat swanga jugupsa parair asamsargah.

[Owing to purity, there is a desire to protect one's own body, being the non-contact with whatever is adverse (to that).]

— *Patanjali Yoga Sutras* ii : 40

SANTOSHA

Santosha, or contentment, is a notion we are all quite familiar with. Ordinarily, human beings experience elation when their incomes unexpectedly rise or they experience a windfall of some type. Yet happiness of this kind is momentary and short-lived. Whether one is rich or poor, whether the Goddess of Fortune smiles on one or not, or whether honor or dishonor comes to one, one should never feel dejected. Keeping the mind focused in a single direction, always being happy, and never feeling regret for any reason, this is the contentment known as *santosha*. If santosha is practiced, unsurpassed joy comes.

Santoshad anuttama sukha labhah.

[Owing to contentment, there is an unexcelled attainment of happiness.]

— *Patanjali Yoga Sutras* ii : 42

TAPAS

Tapas means observances performed to discipline the body and sense organs. According to the *Yoga Yagnavalkya*: "*Vidhinoktena margena Krchra Chandrayanadibih, Sharira Shoshanam prahuh tapasastapa uttamam* [Sages well-versed in austerity say that performing penances such as *krchra* and *chandrayana* (food regulation in accordance with the lunar cycles), which discipline the body in accordance with the scriptures, is the greatest of all the *tapas*)."[14] Thus, *tapas* that follow the injunctions of the *shastras* should be regarded as great.[15] By means of them, impurities are destroyed, the *antah karana* [the inner instrument, made up of mind, intellect, ego, and

---

14 The *Yoga Yagnavalkya* contains the yogic teachings imparted by the ancient sage Yagnavalkya to his student, Gargi.

15 The *shastras* are any sacred texts or books of divine authority, as well as religious and scientific writings.

the faculty of discrimination] becomes purified, and the body and sense organs are perfected.

> Kayendriyasiddhirashuddhiksayah tapasah.
>
> [The perfection of the body and sense organs is due to intensity in spiritual practice, being the elimination of impurities.]
>
> — Patanjali Yoga Sutras ii : 43

SWADHYAYA

Swadhyaya is the recital of Vedic verses and prayers in accordance with strict rules of recitation. Vedic hymns must be recited without damaging the artha [meaning] and Devata [deity] of a mantra through the use of a wrong swara [pitch] or the improper articulation of akshara [letter], pada [word], or varna [sentence].[16]

The Gayatri mantra forms the basis for the study of all Vedic verses, or mantras, which fall into two categories: the Vedic and Tantric.[17] Vedic mantras consist of two types, namely the pragita and apragita, and Tantric mantras, of three types: the strilinga; pullinga; and napumsakalinga. To learn their nature, a text known as the Mantra Rahasya must be studied. However, as mantras such as these are not very helpful to raja yoga, we shall put off discussing them for the time being.[18]

Gods related to the mantras give siddhis [powers] to those who chant them and ponder their meanings, and a Satguru [true or supreme Guru] should be consulted to learn their secrets.

> Swadhyayad ishtadevata samprayogah.
>
> [Owing to the learning and application of personal mantras, there is union with (one's) desired deity.]
>
> — Patanjali Yoga Sutras ii : 44

---

16 In Vedic chanting, there are very strict rules for the recitation of pitch and vowel sounds. To change or mischant a pitch, for example, alters a mantra's meaning. The Devata is the deity embodied in a mantra. Through the correct intonation of a mantra, the deity reveals itself, and its reality is experienced. Thus, in mantras, word, form, and meaning are one, and inextricably connected.

17 The Gayatri is a verse of the sacred Rg Veda addressed to the Sun, and is held to be the holiest passage.

18 In Yoga Mala, raja yoga and ashtanga yoga are treated as synonymous.

Ishwarapranidhana, or surrender to God, means carrying out all our actions, spoken or unspoken, without desiring their fruit, and offering their fruit to the Lord. This is the message of the great sages:

> Kamatah akamatovapi yat karomi shubhashubham
> tat sarvam tvayi vinyasya tvat prayuktah karomyaham.
> [Whatever I do, whether out of desire or not, good or bad,
> having surrendered all that to you, I act as directed by you.]

Such an offering is known as ishwarapranidhana. Through ishwarapranidhana, samadhi [union with the Supreme] is attained, which in turn leads to the attainment of perfection and fulfillment.

> Samadhi Siddih Ishwarapranidhanat.
> [The perfection of samadhi is due to the perfect alignment of
> attention with the omniscient seer within.]
> — Patanjali Yoga Sutras ii : 45

If the limbs and sub-limbs of yama and niyama are to be practiced, then steps should be taken to ensure that one does not fall victim to disease, obligation, or poverty. For when a person becomes ill, his mind cannot be steady, nor can he do any work. Therefore, the body, sense organs, and mind must be stabilized to prevent obstacles, such as disease, from occurring.

To bring the body and sense organs under control, the asanas, or postures, should first be studied and practiced. At various points in the Upanishads, the great sages agree that asana is the first step in the practice of the limbs of yoga:

> Asanam pranasamrodhah pratyaharascha dharanam
> Dhyanam samadhiretani shadangani prakirtita.
> [Asana, pranayama, pratyahara, dharana, dhyana, and samadhi are
> known as the six limbs.]
> — Shandilya Upanishad

Here it has been written that there are but six limbs of yoga, yama and niyama being included under the limbs of pratyahara and dharana. Since the views of Swatmarama and the Upanishadic sages are in agreement on this point, their view is also acceptable to us. It is, after all, not possible to practice the limbs and sub-limbs of *yama* and *niyama* when the body and sense organs are weak and haunted by obstacles. To destroy diseases of the body and sense organs, *asana* must be studied and practiced, which is why Swatmarama speaks of it as the limb to be undertaken first. From its practice, the body will be conditioned and this, in turn, will lead to improved health.

If *asana* is practiced in accordance with established rules, then diseases related to the body and sense organs can be prevented.[19] According to Swatmarama:

> *Hathasya prathamangatvad asanam purvamuchyate*
> *Tasmat asanam kuryat arogyam changalaghavam.*
> [It is said that asana is primary, due to its being the first limb of *hatha* yoga. One should practice that asana which is a state of steadiness, freedom from sickness, and lightness of body.]
> — *Hatha Yoga Pradipika* i : 17

To understand the word *hatha* here, we should know that *ha* means the *surya nadi* and *tha* means the *chandra nadi*. The process of controlling the *prana* [breath] that moves through these two *nadis* is known as *hatha* yoga. Yoga means relation and strength. If the air we breathe through the nostrils is governed by the rules and practice of *pranayama*, or breath control, then the mind will be arrested, as a verse from the *Hatha Yoga Pradipika* affirms:

> *Chale vate chalam chittam*
> *nischale nischalam bhavet.*
> [The breath being in motion, the mind is moving. The breath being without motion, the mind must be motionless.]
> — *Hatha Yoga Pradipika* ii : 2

If, however, our breathing is moving and unregulated, then the mind will be unsteady. Regulating the breathing stabilizes the mind and makes

---

19 The rules here referred to are scriptural instructions.

it firm. The method for directing the stabilized mind toward the Inner Self is what is known as *hatha* yoga.

If the mind moves towards the Self by means of *hatha* yoga, this is known as *raja* yoga. Many people wrongly believe that *hatha* yoga and *raja* yoga are different, but this is not true. As Swatmarama explains in the *Hatha Yoga Pradipika*:

> *Bhrantya bahumatadhvante raja yoga majanatam*
> *Hatha pradipikam dhatte Swatmaramah kripakarah.*
> [Because of the ignorance of the many opinions of those who through error do not understand *raja* yoga, the compassionate Swatmarama offers the *Hatha* Pradipika (the Illumination of *Hatha* Yoga).]
>
> — *Hatha Yoga Pradipika* i : 3

PRANAYAMA

There are many kinds of *pranayama*. Sri Shankara Bhagavadpada speaks of a thousand and explains their methods, while Swatmarama names but eight:

> *Suryabhedanamujjayi sithkari shithali tatha*
> *Bhastrika bhramari murccha plaviniti ashtakumbhakah.*
> [*Suryabedana, ujjayi, sitkari, shitali, bhastrika, bhramari, murchha,* and *plavini* are the eight *kumbhakas.*]
>
> — *Hatha Yoga Pradipika* ii : 44

Of these, only four *pranayamas* are suitable for us.

Some *pranayamas* are useful for curing diseases, some for the purification of the *nadis*, and some for the arrest of the mind. All are important, however, though their practice requires that the preceding step—namely *asana*—be practiced, as well.

If *asana* is practiced, then bodily and sensory diseases will be destroyed. If *pranayama*, conducive to concentrating the mind, strengthening the sense organs, and enabling the mind to be stilled without becoming unstable, is practiced, then diseases present in the body, sense organs, and mind will be cured, allowing the mind to achieve concentration and perceive the Inner Self. Only then will human birth, which results from the penance of many previous lives, be fulfilled, and not by living lives like animals.

In this scientific age, we accept only what we see and reject what we do not. We make no effort to perceive the Universal Self, which is the Indweller that witnesses all actions, that is the cause of the creation, sustenance, and destruction of the universe, and that is of the nature of consciousness. Great scholars and intellectuals who attract attention by using pedantic Vedantic terms which mean that all things are transitory and that only the Supreme Self is real, are only impressing themselves and their listeners for the moment. But soon, the net of delusion is sure to bind them. Therefore, those who want intensely to lift themselves out of the ocean of *samsara*, and to stop wallowing in it and experiencing pleasure and pain, and thereby becoming depressed, should practice yoga, and experience its bliss.[20]

Nothing happens in the world according to our will; that is definite. Everything in the universe occurs in accordance with the will of the Universal Self, not man's desires. If we properly understand the wise gospels of the *Bhagavad Gita*, however, and bring them daily into practice, we will be able to accomplish our goals in life. In no other way can human beings fulfill their wishes. Therefore, performing our dharma and karma free from desire and attachment is our duty.[21] This duty requires us to perform our actions without any worries and to offer all dharma and karma to God, with no expectation of reward. It is difficult to please the Lord by lecturing others on spiritual matters or by attaining popularity or fame. If He is to be pleased, yoga must first be achieved through the relinquishment of the sense of "I" and "mine." From this, we can very shortly attain supreme bliss.

In the *Gita*, the Lord says, "*Purvabhyasena tenaiva hriyate hyavasho'pi sah*," which means that, like a magnet, the mind will be effortlessly attracted to the practice of yoga in this birth by tendencies developed in past births.[22] In other words, if the mind is to develop a love for the prac-

---

20 *Samsara* means the world, mundane existence, and the cycles of birth and re-birth.

21 *Dharma*, in this case, refers to the duties and responsibilities that must be performed as a result of one's station in life; *karma* is one's actions or work.

22 *Bhagavad Gita* vi : 44

tice of yoga, a tendency must already exist from a prior life. Given the earthly and heavenly benefits to be derived from yoga, it would be a great blessing if all people, men and women, were to achieve the practice of the limbs of yoga, which gives happiness both here and hereafter, and is the fulfillment of human experience. This is the noble objective of the author of this book.

Whatever work we attempt cannot be perfectly done unless our minds are tranquil and calm; happiness cannot be attained from it. "*Ashantasya kutah sukham* [For one who is without peace, where is there happiness]?"[23] How can a disturbed mind enjoy comfort? Surely, a human being cannot derive peace and happiness from material objects. Such happiness, even when it does occur, is short-lived, though the suffering that follows is eternal. Disease is the sole consequence of the enjoyment of pleasure, and yoga cannot be attained. Yet yoga liberates us from the devil known as disease. Even *bhoga* [pleasures] become yoga for a mind established in yoga.

If one's mind is impure and overtaken by "I" and "mine," then one's true nature of bliss will be spoiled, and one will become miserable. But the one whose mind is pure will experience eternal bliss. To discover the Inner Self, one should thus practice yoga. Yet, just as a gramophone entertains people by repeating the music sung by others, so too can we attract innocent people by repeating what we have read or heard, and thus win their esteem. When this happens, we soon come to think of ourselves as scholars beyond compare and fall prey to lust and rage. The method for bringing the mind into focus instead and dissolving it in the Atman should be learned under the tutelage of a Guru.[24] Only through the achievement of the yogic limbs, and through the practice of them, can we come to be uplifted—and in no other way.

Focusing the mind in a single direction is extremely important. Since the mind is very unsteady, it is difficult for it to maintain itself in this way. To enable it to stay fixed and in place, *pranayama* is essential. If the breath that moves in and out of the body is arrested, then the mind becomes

---

23 *Bhagavad Gita* ii : 66

24 *Atman*, the Supreme Self, is the all-pervading, self-illumined consciousness.

arrested, as the *Hatha Yoga Pradipika* attests. Thus, the nature of *prana-yama* should be known properly and practiced.

In this world, many things have been created for the pleasure and enjoyment of human beings, and we desire each and every one of them. Yet from these objects of enjoyment come diseases without our desiring them. We should thus know their real nature and develop a detachment from them. By this kind of detachment and by the practice of yoga, our minds will become focused on finding the path to the Supreme Self, whose nature is bliss. When the mind is not attached to things, such as the objects of the senses, it will be able to dissolve itself into the Self. This is what is known as the state of *jivanmukti* [liberation while in the present life].

To be properly learned, *pranayama* must be practiced according to the directions of a Guru. No one should attempt it who thinks that a reading of the scriptures has made him an expert in its knowledge. Rather, an aspirant must carefully learn the rules of *pranayama* first, and avoid haste.

> *Yatha simho gajo vyagro bhavedvashyah shanaih shanaih*
> *Tathaiva sevito vayuranyatha hanti sadhakam.*
> [Just as a lion, elephant or tiger may be gradually brought under control, so is *prana* attended to. Otherwise it destroys the practitioner.]
>
> — *Hatha Yoga Pradipika* ii : 15

In the same way as, with zeal and enterprise, a trainer catches hold of a dangerous animal that wanders the forest freely, such as a tiger, lion, or elephant, and very slowly tames and finally brings it under control, so too will the breath be brought under control, little by little, by the strength of one's practice. Very difficult though this is, it is possible. If, however, an aspirant engages in this practice while violating the rules or with an air of pride and feigned expertise, then he puts himself in danger. Aspirants should bear this fact in mind.

In short, there is no doubt that, through the practice of yoga, one can attain the peace and bliss one desires, the capacity to discriminate between Self and not-Self, peace of mind, and freedom from disease, death, and poverty. A man cannot achieve anything in the world if his sense organs are weak. The experience of the Self, for the weak, is simply not possible.

> Nayam atma balahinena labhyah
> Na medhaya na bahunashrutena.
> [The Self cannot be attained by the weak, by the intellect, or by much learning.]
>
> — Mundaka Upanishad

So say the Vedas. Here the word bala means strength, both physical and mental. The body must be free from diseases of any kind, which divert the mind elsewhere. Physical strength, mental strength, and the strength of the sense organs—all these are very important. Without them, one cannot attain spiritual strength. But intellectual power and a knowledge of the scriptures alone do not lead to Self-realization; the analysis of commentaries and their various explanations do not lead to Self-attainment. Indeed, it is not even enough to study Vedanta at length under the guidance of a Guru.[25] Practice alone is the path to atma labhah [gaining the Self]. The aspirant who follows the precepts and instructions of a Guru with a subdued mind unshackled from the external and internal sense organs, will realize the authentic form of the Universal Self. This is the true nature of yoga.

Body and mind are inseparably related, one to the other. If pleasure and pain are experienced by either the physical body or the sense organs, the mind will experience them as well. This is known to all. If the mind is in pain, the body loses weight, becomes weak and lusterless; if the mind is happy and at peace, the body thrives and develops a strength and luster beyond compare. Hence, the body and sense organs are linked to, and depend upon, the strength of the mind. It is for this reason that the method for concentrating the mind should be known. To learn how to achieve such concentration, the body first must be purified, and then mental strength developed. The method for purifying and strengthening the body is called asana. When the body is purified, the breath also becomes purified, and the diseases of the body are eliminated.

---

25 Vedanta, which literally means the end of the Vedas, is a philosophy of non-dualism.

Once the *asanas* have been learned well enough to be practiced with ease, the next limb to be practiced is that of bringing the breath under control. It is this that is known as *pranayama*. Yet simply sitting, taking in the breath, and letting it out through the nostrils is not *pranayama*. *Pranayama* means taking in the subtle power of the vital wind through *rechaka* [exhalation], *puraka* [inhalation], and *kumbhaka* [breath retention]. Only these *kriyas*, practiced in conjunction with the three *bandhas* [muscle contractions, or locks] and in accordance with the rules, can be called *pranayama*.[26] What are the three *bandhas*? They are *mula bandha*, *uddiyana bandha*, and *jalandhara bandha*, and they should be performed while practicing *asana* and the like.[27] Through the practice of *pranayama*, the mind becomes arrested in a single direction and follows the movement of the breath, a fact known from the scriptural statement *"Chale vate chalam chittam."* It is common knowledge that we lift heavy objects more easily if we hold our breath and concentrate on the objects we are lifting. By controlling the breath through the processes of *rechaka*, *puraka*, and *kumbhaka*, it becomes possible to establish the mind in a single direction.

In *hatha* yoga, there are thousands of methods for *pranayama*. Some purify the *nadis*, others purify and strengthen the body, still others cure diseases and purify the seven *dhatus*, while still others are the means to the knowledge of Brahman through the cessation of the mind.[28] Among these, only the *kumbhaka pranayama*, which is purificatory and useful for Self-realization, is very important. Even *Pujya Shankara Bhagavadpada* calls it the most important of the *pranayamas*:

Sahasrashah santu hatheshu kumbhah sambhavyate kevala kumbha eva.

[Among the *hathas*, there may be a thousandfold *kumbhas*. The pure *kumbha* alone is highly esteemed.]

— *Yoga Taravalli* 10

---

26 A *kriya* is a purification, action or practice.

27 *Mula bandha* [*mula* root : *bandha* lock] means lifting the anus up toward the navel; *uddiyana bandha* [*uddiyana* flying up : *bandha* lock], also known as the stomach lock, means lifting the core muscles four inches below the navel; *jalandhara bandha* means the throat lock.

28 *Ayurvedic* medicine divides the body into seven elements called *dhatus*, which include: lymph and blood plasma; blood; flesh; fat; bone; marrow; and sexual fluids (sperm and ova).

On the subject of *kumbhaka pranayama*, texts such as the *Yoga Yagnavalkya*, *Sutasamhitakara*, *Devi Bhagavata*, *Yoga Vashishtha*, *Bhagavad Gita*, and *Upanishads* follow, on the whole, the opinion of Srimad Acharya Shankara Bhagavadpada. However, because, in general, views about *pranayama* tend to differ, it is important that this yogic limb be learned and practiced under the guidance of a Guru.

For the practitioner of yoga, the rules regarding food, sex, and speech are very important. Among the foods, those called *sattvic* [pure] are the best. Vegetables, however, should not be consumed much. As the Ayurvedic *pramana*, "*Shakena vardate vyadhih* [By vegetables, diseases expand]" and the yoga *pramama* attest, vegetables are unpleasant for practitioners of yoga.[29] Wheat, snake gourd, half-churned curds, mung beans, ginger, milk, and sugar, on the other hand, are best. Indeed, foods that extend the life span; foods that increase *sattvic* qualities, as well as strength, health, happiness, and love; foods that are easily digested; and foods that are natural, genuine, and follow the seasons—these are the most suitable, as they are worthy of being offered to God.

Sour, salty, or spicy foods, on the other hand, are not good for any part of the body and should not be consumed much. If a person's food is pure, then his mind becomes pure, since the mind assumes the qualities of whatever food is consumed, as an Upanishadic authority states: "*Ahara shuddhau sattva shuddih / Sattva shuddhau druvasmrtih* [When the food we take in is pure, our minds become pure / When our minds become pure, memory becomes steady]."[30] The practitioner of yoga should therefore eat only food possessed of *sattvic* qualities. Foods that give rise to passions and mental darkness, or that are fleshy and fattening, should never be consumed, and intoxicating substances, smoking, and the like should also be relinquished.

Only half the stomach should be taken up by the food that is eaten. One quarter of the other half should be given over to water and the remaining quarter left to the movement of air. Consuming too much food or no food at all; sleeping too much or not sleeping at all; having

---

29 *Ayurveda*, which literally means science of life, is the Indian system of living in harmony with ourselves and nature thorough the regulation of our food and activities.

30 *Chandogya Upanishad* vii : 26 : 2

too much sexual intercourse; or mixing with undesirable or uncultured people—all these should be given up as much as possible, as they are obstacles to the practice of yoga. Moderation in regards to eating, sleeping, and the like is thus important to follow.

Similarly, it is not good to talk too much. By talking too much, the power inherent in the tongue decreases and the power of speech is destroyed. When the power of speech is destroyed, our words, too, lose their power, and whatever we utter has no value in society at all. Talk of spiritual matters, however, increases the tongue's power, and is thus helpful to the world. But speech related to mundane matters destroys the power of the tongue, and shortens our life spans. The *shastrakaras* have reflected on and described this fact, so it is better if man follows their path.

Too much sex leads the body, sense organs, and mind to become weak. If the mind and sense organs are weak, we can achieve nothing; our minds grow unsteady and are unable to do anything at all. Therefore, too much sex is to be avoided.

Yoga should neither be practiced in the open air, in a place that is unclean or malodorous, in a basement, nor on a roof. Instead, the place of its practice should be spotlessly clean and level, have windows, and be suitable for smearing with cow dung.[31]

Sweat formed during practice should be wiped dry by rubbing the body with the palms of the hands. If this is done, the body will become lighter and stronger, as a scriptural authority asserts:

> *Jalena shramajatena gatra mardhanam acharet*
> *Drdhatha laghuta chaiva tena gatrasya jayate.*
> [One should practice rubbing the body with the perspiration that comes from exertion. As a result there occurs a firmness and lightness of the body.]
> — Hatha Yoga Pradipika ii : 13

But the body will be sapped and its power exhausted if, in an effort to dry the sweat of practice, it is exposed to the outside air. When this

---

31 In India, cow dung is commonly spread on the ground as a flooring because of the antiseptic qualities it has when it dries.

occurs, a practitioner grows weaker and weaker over time. Thus, the sweat generated by yoga should be gradually dried by rubbing it into the body with the hands, and not by exposing it to the air or by drying it with a towel or cloth. As this is borne out by the experience of yoga practitioners, aspirants should bear it in mind.

The body should not be exposed to the open air for a period of one half hour after practicing. After half an hour, it is good to bathe in hot water. In addition, for the first three months of practice, bathing in cold water and fasting are to be avoided. But, after a practice has become steady and established, these restrictions no longer apply.

During the period of yoga practice, it is advisable to take in much milk and clarified butter, or ghee. Those that cannot afford these should pour a little cold water into some warm cooked rice, mix it together, and eat it before taking any other foods. In this way, the essence that results from using milk and ghee will be generated, and the body will be energized and nourished.

Aspirants should be mindful to follow the above-mentioned rules regarding food, sexual habits, bathing, and practice. They should also be devoted to God and Guru. Practicing yoga for the sake of one's health, a firm body, or enjoyment is not the right approach. Only the purification of the body, sense organs, and mind, and the dedication of all actions and deeds to the Almighty, is the true way. If our minds are offered to the Supreme Self in this way, our hopes and aspirations will be fulfilled by Him at the appropriate times. Aspirants should thus guard against those things that would disrupt their mental equilibrium.

To be able to practice yoga, one must possess enthusiasm, zeal, courage, and a firm faith in *tattvajnana* [philosophical knowledge]. One should also not mingle with the crowd. With these qualities, an aspirant can attain yoga. Yogis describe the path to yogic attainment in this way:

> *Utsahatsahasadhaivyattattvajnansh cha nischayat*
> *Janasanghaparityagat shadbiryogah prasiddhyate.*
> [By means of enthusiasm, boldness, firmness, discrimination of truth, conviction, and the avoidance of public gatherings, by these six things, is yoga accomplished.]
> — *Hatha Yoga Pradipika* i : 16

Aspirants should learn the rules outlined above. They should not listen to, nor become discouraged by, the words of those who have no knowledge of yogic practice, or who are too lethargic to bring their own bodies under control.

There is no age limit for the practice of yoga and it can be practiced by anyone—by women, men, the weak, and by those who are sick or disabled—as the *shastrakaras* affirm:

> *Yuva vrddho'thivrddho va vyadhito durbalo'pi va*
> *Abhyasat siddimapnoti sarvayogeshvatandritah.*
> [Whether young, old or very old, sick or debilitated, one who is vigilant attains success in all the yogas, by means of practice.]
> — Hatha Yoga Pradipika i : 64

Thus do the experts give their unanimous approval to this idea, and experience also confirms it. Indeed, only lazy people find the practice of the yogic limbs useless. Otherwise, yoga is very important for anyone eight years or older, regardless of sex.

Pregnant women who have crossed into the fourth month should abstain from doing *asanas*. They can, however, practice *ujjayi pranayama*, *samavritti pranayama*, and *vishamavritti pranayama*, without *kumbhaka*, until the seventh month. In this way, if they regularly practice deep *rechaka*, or exhalation, and *puraka*, or inhalation, while sitting in *Padmasana* [lotus posture] or *Mahamudra* [the great seal], they will have a smoother and easier delivery. It is good for women to keep this in mind.

For people over fifty, it is enough to practice some of the easier and more useful *asanas*, as well as some of the *pranayamas*. Those who have been practicing for many years, however, can do any *asana* or *pranayama* without a problem. Older people who want to start yoga, however, will find practicing the following ten *asanas* sufficient [see Chapter 2 for detailed descriptions of individual *asanas*]: first, the *Surya Namaskara* (types 1 and 2); then *Paschimattanasana*; *Sarvangasana*; *Halasana*; *Karnapidasana*; *Urdhva Padmasana*; *Pindasana*; *Matsyasana*; *Uttana Padasana*; and *Shirshasana*. It is preferable to do these in concert with the *vinyasas* [breathing and movement systems], but if this is not possible, then practicing while focusing on *rechaka* and *puraka* will suffice.

Shirshasana should be practiced for at least ten minutes, and the rest, for at least ten *rechaka* and *puraka* while in the state of the *asana* [*see fn. 39*]. By practicing in this way, the body and sense organs will become firm, the mind purified, longevity will be increased, and the body will be filled with fresh energy.

For the middle-aged, it is best to do all the *asanas*. The more they are practiced, the stronger the body becomes, and obstacles such as disease cease to be a problem. *Pranayama* is easier, the mind becomes more harmonious as the quality of *sattva* [purity] comes to predominate, and intellectual power and longevity are augmented.

For the very old, however, who find the practice of *Sarvangasana*, *Halasana*, *Uttana Padasana*, *Shirshasana*, and *Padmasana* too difficult, it is enough to practice *mahabandha* daily, as well as *rechaka kumbhaka pranayama*, *puraka kumbhaka pranayama*, *samavritti vishamavritti pranayama*, and *sithali pranayama*. These will help them live happier and longer lives, and will insulate them from disease.

The weak and the sick, too, should gradually practice suitable *asanas* and *pranayamas*, and over time, as their strength increases, their practices should also increase. In this way, the diseases of the sick and the strengthlessness of the weak will be eliminated, leaving them healthy and vigorous.

The aspirant that goes to a Guru will find that the Guru will tailor his practice to his particular bodily constitution. Yoga should never be learned from reading books or looking at pictures. It should only be learned under the guidance of a Guru who knows the yogic science and is experienced in its practice. If this is ignored, it is possible for physical and mental problems to occur. For while it is true that all the diseases that afflict the body and mind of a human being can be eliminated by the practice of the limbs of yoga, it is also true that this will only occur if the science is brought into practice under an experienced Guru who knows the yoga *shastra* properly and who implements it in practice. Only in this way can the body, mind, and senses be purified, just as gold is in a crucible.

Through the practice of yoga, many types of incurable ailments, such as asthma, can be cured, and the body, mind, and senses will come to radiate with new energy. Indeed, some physicians who condemn the science of yoga have been dumbfounded to find former patients of theirs being cured of their diseases by yoga. This is borne out by experience. Diseases that cannot be cured by medicine can be cured by yoga; diseases that cannot be cured by yoga cannot be cured at all. That is definite. A doctor can find remedies for illnesses that result from an imbalance of the three *doshas*, but no *dhanvanthari* [doctor dealing in medicine] has a remedy to offer for mental illness.[32] Yet yogis say that even for this, there is a yogic cure. Indeed, the practitioner that keeps faith in and practices the limbs of yoga can achieve anything in the world. He can even redo creation.[33]

The world is full of falsehood, deceit, and exploitation. A yogi has the power to correct this and to attract people of the world to the right path. It is therefore necessary to stress again the importance of practitioners of yoga keeping faith in, and showing devotion to, the yogic limbs and the Guru. But neither faith in nor devotion to the Guru is common among young people today. The weakness of the mind and sense organs accounts for this. And yet knowledge learned without devotion to God and Guru is like pouring the milk of a sacred cow into a bag of dog's skin, or the undrinkable milk of a donkey's udder. But if young men and women genuinely pursue knowledge, practice true faith and devotion, and do not yield to mental unsteadiness or sham piety, then the divine power will confer knowledge on them in abundance—knowledge which will make them theists of firm bodies and strong minds who are freed from lust and the like; there is no doubt about it. There is also no doubt that a country privileged enough to have the majority of its young people be possessed of minds devoted to God, in addition to firm bodies and mental power, will be blessed with bounty. This is on Vedic authority. Thus, let it be emphasized again that if practitioners know the path described above, and practice it, they will attain happiness here as well as hereafter.

As the bodily constitution of each human being is different, it is important to practice the *asanas* accordingly. The benefit to be had from

---

32 *Vata* [wind], *pitta* [fire, bile], and *kapha* [earth, phlegm] are the three *doshas*, which are functional elements responsible for each and every activity of the body and which are excited by food and actions. When the *doshas* are in harmony, there is health; when there is disharmony among them, disease follows.

33 In demonstration of this, Vishvamitra, a great *rishi* [seer], created another *Indra Loka* [world of the Gods] for a low-caste man who wanted to go to Heaven.

one *asana* or *pranayama* can be derived just as well from another that better suits the structure of a person's body. Some *asanas* are not suitable for particular people and may be painful. A Guru will understand this and be able to explain it, so the practitioner of yoga must be certain to follow his guidance.

To begin the practice of yoga, an aspirant should first do the *Surya Namaskara* [Sun Salutations], and then proceed to the *asanas*. The *Surya Namaskara* and *asanas* must be practiced in the correct sequence and follow the method of *vinyasa*. If they are not, or the movement of *rechaka* and *puraka* is neglected, no part of the body will become strong, the subtle *nadis* will not be purified, and, owing to the resulting imbalance, the body, sense organs, mind, and intellect will not develop. They may even come to be further imbalanced.

If the *asanas* and the *Surya Namaskara* are to be practiced, they must be done so in accordance with the prescribed *vinyasa* method only. As the sage Vamana says, "*Vina vinyasa yogena asanadin na karayet* [O yogi, do not do *asana* without *vinyasa*]."[34] When yoga is practiced with a knowledge of its proper method, it is quite easy to learn, but practiced without such knowledge, it becomes a very difficult undertaking. Therefore, aspirants should not forget to learn the method of *vinyasa*, as well as of *rechaka* and *puraka*, and to follow it in their practice.

The *asanas* described in the next chapter belong to the curative aspect of yogic practice. They will be discussed systematically, and aspirants should be careful to practice them in the order in which they are described, and not to skip one posture in preference for another. This must be borne in mind.

Winter is the best time of year to start yoga and an aspirant should practice before five o'clock in the morning. Warming up by the fire or by jogging during the winter is to be avoided, however, as is too much sexual intercourse. These are things an aspirant should not forget.

> *Stirairangais tushtuvagumsastanubhih*
> *Vyashema devahitam yaddayuh*
> *Om Shanti Shanti Shanti.*

---

34 Vamana is the author of *Yoga Korunta*, the authoritative text on *asana* and *pranayama* in *ashtanga* yoga.

[While praising, may we of strong and steady limb
enjoy the life given by the Gods
Om Peace Peace Peace.]

— *Shanti Mantra* from the *Ṛg Veda*

Surya Namaskara
and
Yoga Asanas

Surya Namaskara

THE PRACTICE OF THE SURYA NAMASKARA, OR SUN SALUTATIONS, HAS COME down to us from the long distant past, and is capable of rendering human life heavenly and blissful. By means of it, people can become joyous, experience happiness and contentment, and avoid succumbing to old age and death.[35]

Yet, nowadays, without ever having learned the traditions and practices of their ancestors and having no control over their sense organs, people engage in self-indulgence and destroy their mental powers for the sake of tangible gain. They deny reality simply because it cannot be seen and make their lives miserable, or subject to disease, poverty, and death. If they were to follow the traditions of their ancestors, however, they would develop their bodies and minds, and, in so doing, make possible the realization of the nature of the Self, as a scriptural authority confirms: "*Nayam atma balahinena labhyah* [This Self cannot be gained by one devoid of strength]."[36] With strengthened bodies, sense organs, and minds, they would become healthy and righteous, live long and intellectual lives, and be able to attain eternal liberation. Thus, if we want lives of health, righteousness, intellectuality, and longevity, let us never forget the ways and traditions of our ancestors.

By following the precept of the great sages, "*Shariramadyam khalu dharma Sadhanam* [The first duty is to take care of the body, which is the means to the pursuit of spiritual life]," our ancestors found the means to bodily health.[37] Such means, they knew, should not violate the scriptures, but be in accordance with them. And this, they knew, could only be possible through the *Surya Namaskara* and limbs of yoga. So they studied yogic science, brought it into practice, and were joyful. In all corners of India, too, people of every class were bringing the *Surya Namaskara* described in the yoga *shastra* into practice. This they did with the feeling that they were performing a righteous action which was a daily duty, for they knew the blessings of the Sun God are essential to good health. If we

---

35 It is said that, for the greatest yogis, it is even possible to have power over death, as life can be extended by controlling the breath.

36 *Mundaka Upanishad* iii : 2 : 3

37 *Meditation and Spiritual Life*, Swami Yatishwarananda, Ramakrishna Ashram pub., Bangalore.

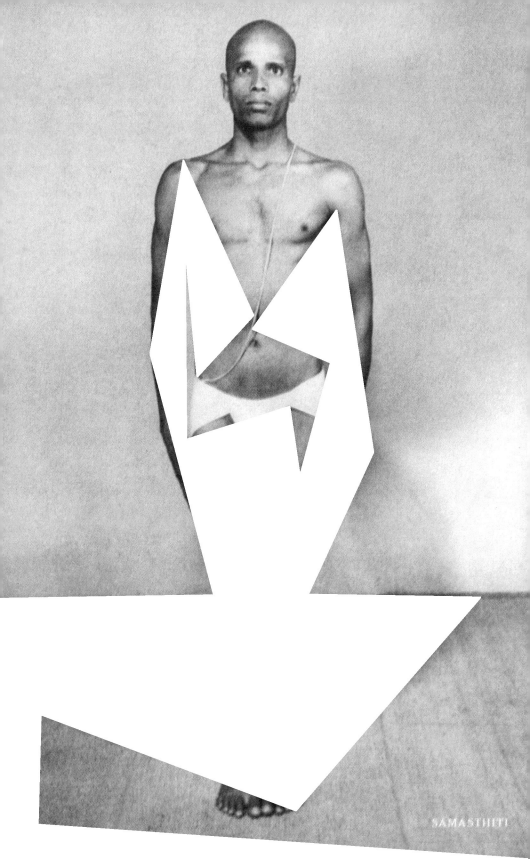

SAMASTHITI

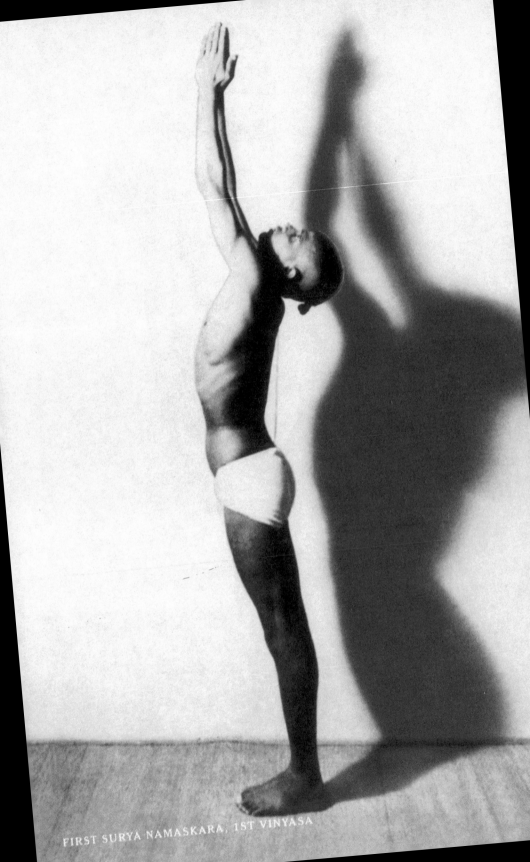

FIRST SURYA NAMASKARA, 1ST VINYASA

reflect on the saying "*Arogyam bhaskarad icchet* [One should desire health from the sun]," it is clear that those blessed by the Sun God live healthy lives. Therefore, for health—the greatest wealth of all—to be attained, the blessings of the Sun God must alone be sought.

To secure these blessings, the *Surya Namaskara* should be practiced in accordance with scriptural rules. The worship of the Sun must always be in the *Namaskara* form, since, while there are other forms of worship, the *Namaskara* alone are important. In the words of the scripture: "*Namaskarapriya suryah* [*Namaskara* is the beloved of the sun]." Thus, they should not be practiced whimsically, but in accordance with the method prescribed in the *shastra*. For it is only by the *Namaskara*, done in consonance with the rules and without violating the scripture, that the Sun, the God associated with health, will be pleased and confer the wealth of vitality upon us, and protect us as well. In short, if a person is to secure the fortune of health, he should perform the *Surya Namaskara* without abandoning the path prescribed in the *shastras*.

What are the *shastras*? They explain the meaning of mantras in such a way that even dull minds can easily understand them. Among the *shastras*, those that elucidate the import of mantras related to the Sun God offer adorations and prayers to Him as follows: "*Bhadram karnebhih shrunuyama devah / Bhadram pashyema / Akshabhir yajatrah* [O Gods, while engaged in sacrifices, may we hear with our ears what is auspicious, may we see with our eyes what is auspicious]." The purport of this mantra is to discern divinity in all the objects of the senses through the strengthening of the senses. It is a prayer not merely for the strength of the body, senses, and the mind, and for the elimination of diseases, but for inner happiness and ultimate liberation from transmigratory existence. If such happiness is to be gained, it can only be so by the healthy, not by the sick. Therefore, to become healthy, one should practice the *Surya Namaskara* in accordance with scriptural injunctions.

The method for doing the *Surya Namaskara* has been described in various ways by various people. We cannot categorically state which is correct, but when we reflect on the science of yoga, we see that the tradition of the *Surya Namaskara* follows, in the main, the method of *vinyasa*, or breathing and movement system, the movements of *rechaka*, or exhalation, *puraka*, or inhalation, and meditation. According to the

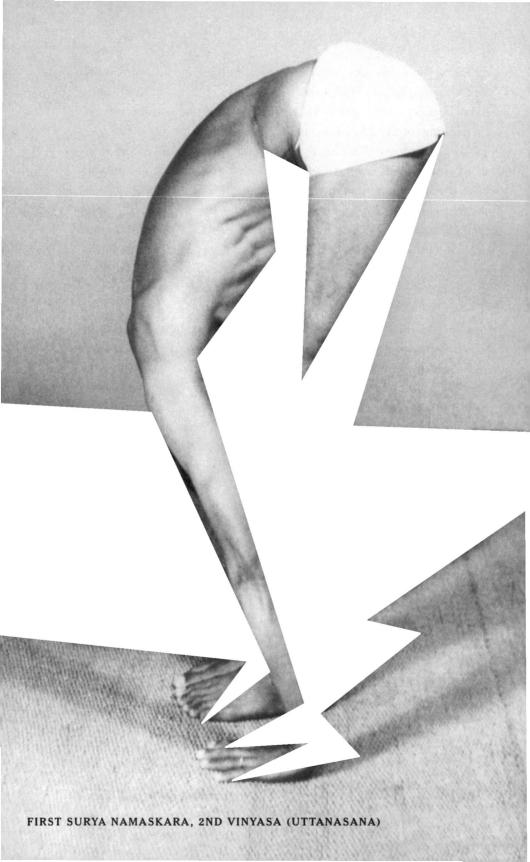

FIRST SURYA NAMASKARA, 2ND VINYASA (UTTANASANA)

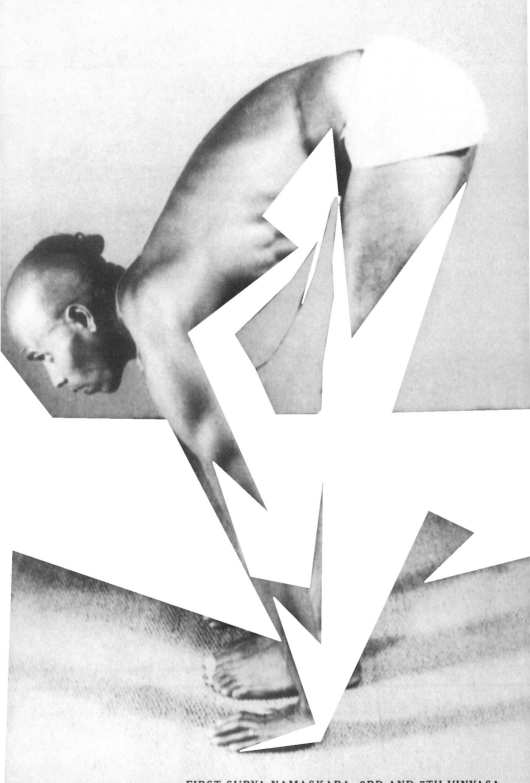

FIRST SURYA NAMASKARA, 3RD AND 7TH VINYASA

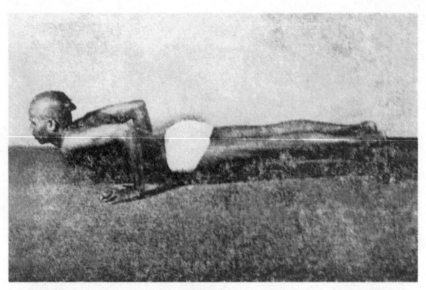

FIRST SURYA NAMASKARA, 4TH VINYASA; SECOND SURYA NAMASKARA, 8TH AND
12TH VINYASA (CHATURANGA DANDASANA)

yoga *shastra*, this tradition includes: *vinyasa; rechaka* and *puraka; dhyana*
[meditation]; *drishti* [sight, or gazing place]; and the *bandhas* [muscle contractions, or locks]. And this alone is the method which should be followed
when learning the *Surya Namaskara*, as yogis declare from experience.
Indeed, the Sun Salutations done without following the rules mentioned
above are little more than exercise, and not true *Surya Namaskara*.

There are two types of *Surya Namaskara*. The first consists of nine
vinyasas, and the second, of seventeen. To learn the method for the
vinyasas, rechaka and *puraka*, the *bandhas, dhyana*, and for *trataka* [gazing]
and the like, one should be certain to consult a *Satguru*, for it would be
wrong to try to learn yoga without recourse to such a teacher. If, however, one follows the scriptural path, and brings it into practice under the
guidance of a *Satguru* who is not only well-versed in the yoga *shastra* but
who has brought it into practice himself, then the three-fold diseases will
be destroyed, and one will live a healthy life.[38]

There is a common perception that no medicine exists for mental ill-

---

38 The three-fold diseases are: *manasika*, or mental; *desika*, or bodily; and *adhyatmika*, or spiritual.

ness. The *Shrutis*, however, say that through the *Surya Namaskara*, even mental illness can be cured. Now, if we reflect on the meaning of a mantra such as: "*Hridrogyam mama surya harimanam cha nashaya* [Remove, O Sun, the pallor unhealthy to my heart and mind]," we see that even mental illnesses and diseases born of *prarabdha karma* [the results of past actions that are bearing fruit in this lifetime] can be destroyed. Our ancestors certainly studied the mantras, understood their meanings, and put them into practice. As a result, they lived long lives of good health, great strength, and high intellect, and, without ever succumbing to disease, death, or poverty, they attained divine knowledge, merged with bliss, and were forever content.

Thus, if the scriptural way of practicing the *Surya Namaskara* is followed, the most terrible diseases, such as leprosy, epilepsy, and jaundice, will be cured. In this regard, no one need entertain any doubt or disbelief; without question, the terrible diseases just referred to can be destroyed. Some people have received medical treatment for illnesses such as leprosy for years without ever being cured. Within five to six months, however, of practicing the *Surya Namaskara*, *yogasana*, *pranayama*, and the like, they have found themselves relieved of their ailments. This is borne out by my own experience. Therefore, people who practice yoga and the *Surya Namaskara* will not fall victim to maladies of any type. Hence, aspirants should engage in their practice and leave behind all fear and doubt.

Some people work by sitting or standing in one place for long periods of time and experience pains in their joints which make them unable to sit or walk without great difficulty. They pursue all kinds of medical treatment, and lead futile lives. But their afflictions can definitely be cured by the *Surya Namaskara*. Yogis speak of such afflictions as being associated with the *nadis*. To keep the body, which is the foundation of the performance of all sorts of meritorious deeds, pure and free from obstacles such as disease as much as possible, the *Surya Namaskara* and *yogasana* are very important. Indeed, in the present world, they are essential to all, men and women, young and old. Were all people to recognize their usefulness, bring them into practice, and teach their traditions to their families, it can be said with pride that our holy land of India would rejoice to find itself filled with fresh energy. Were the government itself

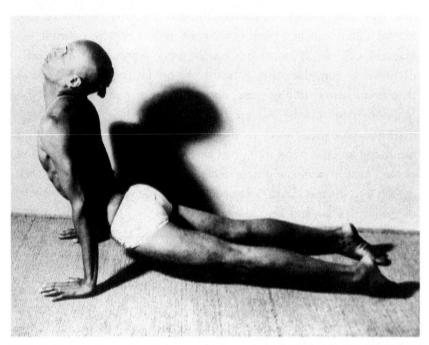

FIRST SURYA NAMASKARA, 5TH VINYASA; SECOND SURYA NAMASKARA, 9TH AND 13TH VINYASA
(URDHVA MUKHA SVANASANA)

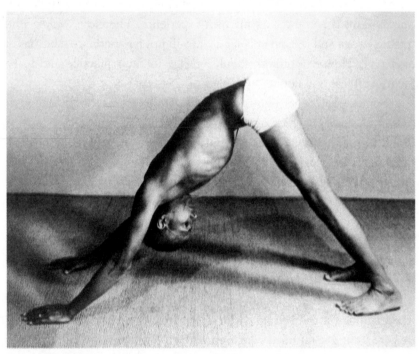

FIRST SURYA NAMASKARA, 6TH VINYASA; SECOND SURYA NAMASKARA, 10TH AND 14TH VINYASA
(ADHO MUKHA SVANASANA)

to understand their usefulness, and make the practice of *yogasana*, the *Surya Namaskara*, and their traditions compulsory for all students in all educational institutions, boys and girls alike, which would help to render their lives pure, it would be doing a great service to the world. Indeed, Mother India would be very pleased. We should, therefore, never forget to carry the torch of this divine light of yogic knowledge, which has been passed down to us with our Vedic culture, and to keep its flame alight for all eternity.

METHOD FOR DOING THE FIRST SURYA NAMASKARA

The first type of *Surya Namaskara* has nine *vinyasas*. To begin, join the legs together, with the heels and big toes touching, push the chest up, lower the head slightly, and stand straight, gazing at the tip of the nose; this is called *Samasthiti*, which means standing up in a straight line. Then, taking the breath in slowly through the nose, raise the arms straight up over the head, bring the hands together, lean the head back a little, and look at the fingertips; this is the 1st *vinyasa*. Then, releasing the breath slowly, bring the hands down to the floor on either side of the feet, straighten the knees, and touch the knees slowly with the nose; this is the 2nd *vinyasa* (*see figure*). Then, doing *puraka* (which means inhaling), lift only the head; this is the 3rd *vinyasa*. (*For all subsequent* vinyasas, *see figures*.) Next, doing *rechaka* (which means exhaling), press the hands squarely onto the floor and, with only the strength of the hands, throw the legs back and hold the body straight on the hands and toes only; this is the 4th *vinyasa*. Then, doing *puraka*, push the chest forward with the strength of the hands, lift the head up, bend the waist, straighten the arms without touching either the thighs or knees to the floor, and extend the feet, toes pointed and tops pressed to the floor; this is the 5th *vinyasa*. For all the *vinyasas*, the body should be kept tight and straight. Then, doing *rechaka*, lift the waist up, tilt the head under, press the heels to the floor, pull in the stomach completely, and hold position, gazing at the navel; this is the 6th *vinyasa*. Following this, the 7th *vinyasa* conforms to the method of the 3rd *vinyasa*, meaning that while moving from the 6th *vinyasa* to the 7th *vinyasa*, do *puraka*, jump the feet in between the hands, press the legs together, and stand with the knees straightened and feet joined. The 8th *vinyasa* then follows the method of the 2nd *vinyasa*, and

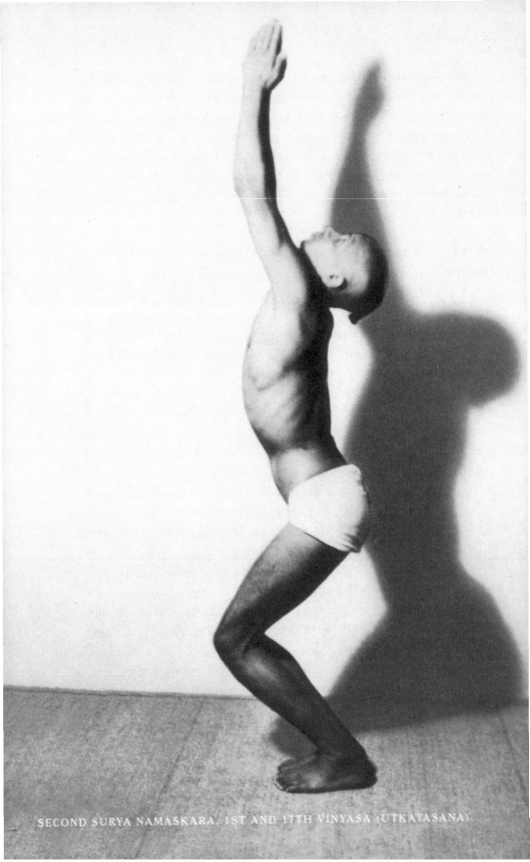

SECOND SURYA NAMASKARA, 1ST AND 17TH VINYASA (UTKATASANA)

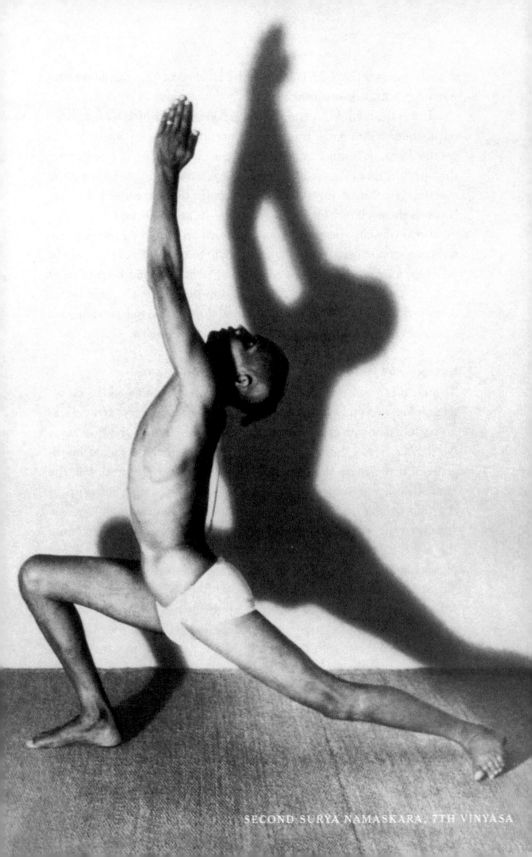

SECOND SURYA NAMASKARA, 7TH VINYASA

the 9th *vinyasa* follows the method of the 1st *vinyasa*. One should then be standing up straight in *Samasthiti*.

This is the method for the first *Surya Namaskara*, which is often practiced while chanting mantras. For this, meditation is very important, as are the *drishti*, or gazing places, which include: *nasagra drishti* [the gaze on the tip of the nose] for *samasthiti; broomadhya drishti* [the gaze between the eyebrows] for the 1st *vinyasa; nasagra dristri* for the 2nd *vinyasa*; the gaze between the eyebrows for the 3rd *vinyasa*—in other words, for the odd-numbered *vinyasas*, the gaze should be focused between the eyebrows and, for the even-numbered ones, the gaze should be on the tip of the nose. In addition, for the even-numbered *vinyasas, rechaka* should be performed and, for the odd, one should do *puraka*. On the whole, the method for doing *rechaka* and *puraka* is the same for all the *vinyasas* and *asanas* ahead. A *sadhaka* [spiritual aspirant] should learn it with patience.

METHOD FOR DOING THE SECOND SURYA NAMASKARA

The second type of *Surya Namaskara* has seventeen *vinyasas* and its movements of *rechaka* and *puraka* are the same as for the first *Surya Namaskara*. To begin, stand straight, joining the legs together, as in the first *Surya Namaskara*. Then, doing *puraka*, bend the knees, which should be together, lift the chest, raise the arms straight up over the head, join the hands together, lean the head back a little, and stand gazing at the tips of the fingers; this is the 1st *vinyasa (see figure)*. Next, doing *rechaka*, straighten the legs (do not bend the knees), press the hands down onto the floor on either side of the feet, as described in the first *Surya Namaskara*, and touch the knees with the nose; this is the 2nd *vinyasa*. Then, doing *puraka*, straighten the back, lift the head only; this is the 3rd *vinyasa*. Next, doing *rechaka* slowly, jump the body back into the form of a stick with only the strength of the hands, as described in the first *Surya Namaskara*, and rest with the head lifted a little; this is the 4th *vinyasa*. Then, doing *puraka*, push the body forward with the force of the arms, lift the chest, arch the back, and make the legs tight and straight, resting with the tops of the feet pressed to the floor; this is the 5th *vinyasa*. Then, doing *rechaka*, lift the waist up, press the heels to the floor, tilt the head, draw in the stomach tightly, and stare at the navel; this is the 6th *vinyasa*. Next, doing *puraka*, place the right foot between the hands, which are pressed to the floor, bend the knee of the right leg, straighten the thigh and knee of the left leg which is stretched back, raise the arms straight up over the head, bring the hands together, swell the chest, lean the head back a little, and rest, staring at the tips of the fingers; this is the 7th *vinyasa (see figure)*. The 8th *vinyasa* then follows the method of the 4th *vinyasa*. The 9th *vinyasa* follows the method of the 5th *vinyasa*. The 10th *vinyasa* follows the method of the 6th. The 11th *vinyasa* follows the method of the 7th, though for the 7th *vinyasa*, the right leg comes forward and, in the 11th *vinyasa*, the left leg comes forward; this should be noted. Then, the 12th *vinyasa* again follows the method of the 4th. The 13th *vinyasa* follows the method of the 5th. The 14th *vinyasa* follows the method of the 6th. The 15th *vinyasa* follows the method of the 3rd. The 16th *vinyasa* follows the method of the 2nd, and the 17th *vinyasa* follows the method of the 1st. Then, comes *Samasthiti*.

For the second *Surya Namaskara*, the *vinyasas*, *rechaka*, and *puraka* follow the method described in the first *Surya Namaskara*. The only difference is that, in the second *Surya Namaskara*, the 1st, 7th, 11th, and 17th *vinyasas* introduce a different form; otherwise, the remaining *vinyasas* are the same as those for the first Sun Salutation. As earlier noted, even-numbered *vinyasas* indicate *rechaka*, and those with odd numbers signal *puraka*.

Aspirants should know this method, which is best learned from a Guru. They should also note that *kumbhaka*, or breath retention, does not occur either in the *Surya Namaskara* or the *asanas*. Those who practice the *Surya Namaskara* in accordance with scriptural rules must never forget to be mindful of the *drishti*, *bandhas*, *dhyana*, *rechaka*, and *puraka*, as discussed earlier. After finishing the Sun Salutations, worship and other religious activities should be performed while sitting in *Padmasana*. For those who practice *asanas*, the *Surya Namaskara* must be performed first and then followed by the *asanas*. This is the rule. Those who follow this rule will receive whatever they desire.

With this, the topic of the *Surya Namaskara* comes to a close.

Yoga Asanas

The *asanas* that follow the *Surya Namaskara* should be
practiced in the manner described below.

1. Padangushtasana

Padangushtasana has three *vinyasas*, of which the 2nd is the state of the
asana (see figure).[39]

METHOD

First, stand up straight, inhaling through the nostrils deeply, jump the legs
apart as much as half a foot, slowly let the breath out, reach down and
take hold of the big toes, lift the head and chest up completely without
bending the knees, and stay in position while inhaling; this is the 1st
vinyasa. Then, letting the breath out, take in the lower abdomen, place
the head in the region between the two knees, straighten the knees, and
stay in position, doing *puraka* and *rechaka* as much as possible; this is the
2nd *vinyasa (see figure).*[40] Next, inhaling, slowly lift the head, remaining
in position with the fingers holding the big toes; this is the 3rd *vinyasa.*
Then exhale and return to *Samasthiti.* While in the state of this *asana,* the
lower abdomen should be drawn in and held tightly, and *rechaka* and
puraka should be done slowly and as much as possible. This is the way to
do *Padangushtasana.*

BENEFITS

Padangushtasana dissolves the fat of the lower abdomen, and purifies both
the *kanda,* or egg-shaped nerve plexus in the anal region, and the rectum.

2. Padahastasana

Padahastasana has three *vinyasas.* The 2nd *vinyasa* is the state of the *asana.*

---

39 The state of an *asana* refers to the key position of a posture.
40 Note: Throughout the descriptions of the *asanas,* breathing instructions are given which direct
aspirants to do *rechaka* and *puraka,* or exhale and inhale, as much as possible. It is sufficient, however, to breathe in and out five to eight times in each posture. To remedy a particular ailment, an
aspirant may remain in the curative postures specific to a complaint for 50 to 80 breaths.

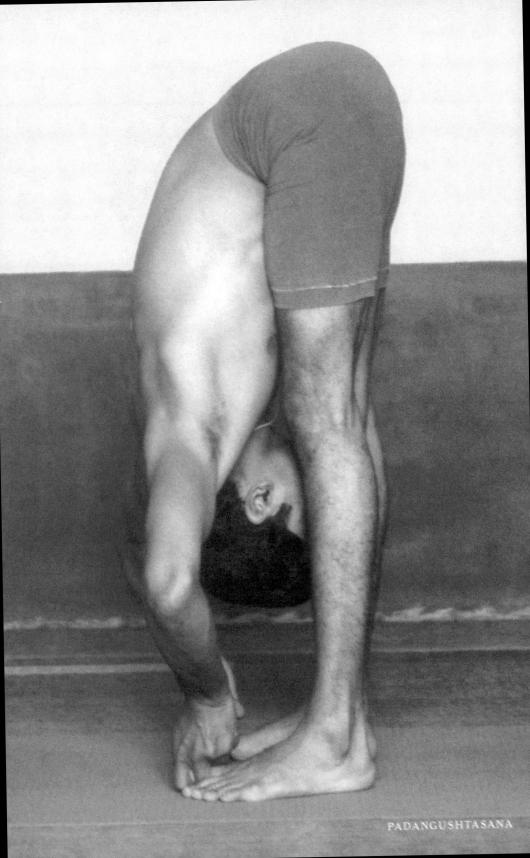

PADANGUSHTASANA

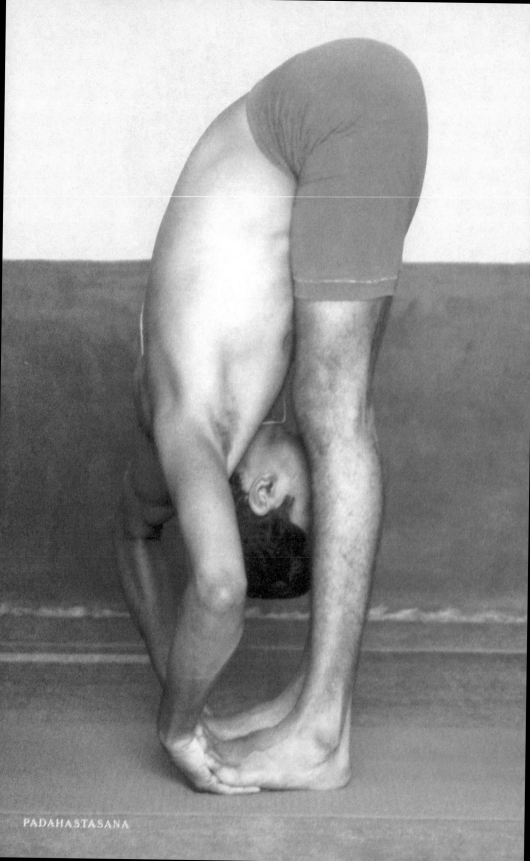

PADAHASTASANA

To begin, stand with the legs as much as half a foot apart, as in *Padangushthasana*, and doing *puraka* and then *rechaka*, place palms under the feet and, doing *puraka*, lift the head up and stay in position; this is the 1st *vinyasa*. Then, doing *rechaka*, place the head in the region between the knees, keeping knees straight, and hold position, doing *rechaka* and *puraka* fully as much as possible; this is the 2nd *vinyasa*. Then, taking the breath in, lift only the head; this is the 3rd *vinyasa*. Then *Samasthiti*, as in the earlier *asana*. In the state of this *asana*, the lower abdomen should be drawn in tightly, and *rechaka* and *puraka* done as much as possible.

BENEFITS

Padahastasana purifies the anal canal, kidneys, and lower abdomen.

3. UTTHITA TRIKONASANA

Utthita Trikonasana has five *vinyasas*, of which the 2nd and 4th are the states of the *asana*. *Rechaka* and *puraka* should be performed as above and, as with the *Surya Namaskara*, *rechaka* occurs in the even-numbered *vinyasas* and *puraka* in the odd. Aspirants should note the correct movements of both, and perform them properly.

METHOD

First, beginning with *puraka*, jump the legs open to the right, three feet apart, stretch the arms out wide on either side of the torso at chest level, and hold; this is the 1st *vinyasa*. Then, turn the right foot to the right and exhaling, reach down and take hold of the big toe of the right foot with the right hand, lift up the other arm, fix the gaze on its fingertips, and do *puraka* and *rechaka* slowly and as much as possible; this is the 2nd *vinyasa*; for this *vinyasa*, both knees must be kept straight (*see figure*.) Then, doing *puraka*, return to the position of the 1st *vinyasa*, and hold; this is the 3rd *vinyasa*. Then, turn the left foot to the left, and doing *rechaka*, reach down and take hold of the big toe, gaze at the tip of the raised hand, and do *puraka* and *rechaka* as much as possible; this is the 4th *vinyasa*. Then, doing *puraka*, return to the position of the 1st *vinyasa*; this is the 5th *vinyasa*. Then, return to *Samasthiti*.

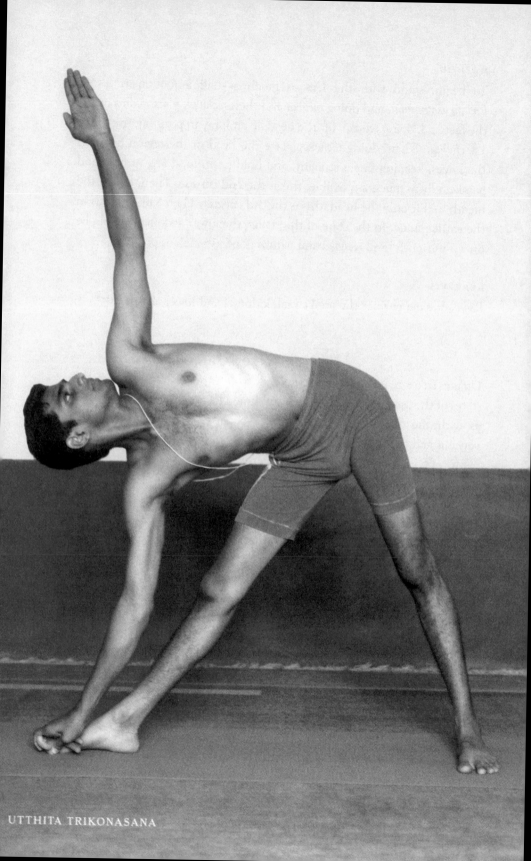

UTTHITA TRIKONASANA

Utthita Trikonasana dissolves the bad fat at the waist, and brings the body into shape. It also expands the narrow portion of the breathing channel and strengthens the backbone.

4. Utthita Parshvakonasana

This *asana* has five *vinyasas*, of which the 2nd and 4th constitute the states of the *asana* (*see figure*). *Rechaka* and *puraka* should follow the method described for earlier *asanas*.

METHOD

For this *asana*, jump the legs open to the right, doing *puraka*, and stand with the legs as much as five feet apart, as in *Trikonasana*, stretching out the arms tightly at the level of the chest, and swelling the chest. Then, doing *rechaka*, turn the right foot out, bend the knee completely, place the right hand by the side of the right foot, stretch the left arm straight out over the ear, and gaze at the fingertips; this is the 2nd *vinyasa*, which is the state of the *asana* and during which *puraka* and *rechaka* should be done as much as possible. Then, doing *puraka*, return to the position of the 1st *vinyasa*; this is the 3rd *vinyasa*. Then, as with the right leg and doing *rechaka*, repeat above for the left leg; this is the 4th *vinyasa*. Next, doing *puraka*, return to the position of the 1st *vinyasa*; this is the 5th *vinyasa*. Then come to *Samasthiti*.

In the 2nd and 4th *vinyasas*, which are the states of this *asana*, the body should be held tightly, and *rechaka* and *puraka* done slowly and as much as possible. Indeed, in whatever *asana*, aspirants should not forget to perform *rechaka* and *puraka* slowly and as much as possible while in the *asana's* state.

BENEFITS

Utthita Parshvakonasana purifies the ribs and lower abdomen, dissolves the bad fat at the waist, and softens the limbs so that subsequent *asanas* can be more easily practiced.

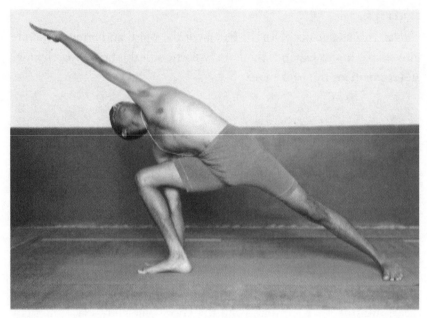

UTTHITA PARSHVAKONASANA

5. Prasarita Padottanasana (A)

This four-part *asana* has five *vinyasas*, of which the 3rd is the state of the *asana*. In the 2nd *vinyasa*, aspirants should note that both *rechaka* and *puraka* are to be performed.

METHOD

Jump to the right, doing *puraka* and spreading the legs as much as five feet apart, as in *Utthita Parshvakonasana*, and place the hands on the waist; this is the 1st *vinyasa*. Then, doing *rechaka*, press the hands to the floor with the fingertips in line with the big toes, keeping the head lifted and doing *puraka* slowly; this is the 2nd *vinyasa*. Next, doing *rechaka*, place the head on the floor between the hands, keeping the legs straight and tight, and hold position with waist lifted, doing *puraka* and *rechaka* as much as possible; this is the 3rd *vinyasa*, during which the stomach should be drawn in properly, using only the *uddiyana bandha*, or stomach lock, and by slightly loosening the *mula bandha*, or anal lock *(see figure)*. Then, doing *puraka*, lift and hold the head up completely, and do *rechaka*; this is the 4th *vinyasa*. Next, doing *puraka*, lift the hands and place them on the waist, and return to the position of the 1st *vinyasa*; this is the 5th *vinyasa*. Then follows *Samasthiti*.

PRASARITA PADOTTANASANA (B)

This is the second part of *Prasarita Padottanasana*. *Rechaka* and *puraka* should be performed as above.

METHOD

Doing *puraka*, stand, as in *Prasarita Padottanasana* (A), stretch arms out to the sides at chest level and straighten them, as in *Trikonasana*, and hold position; this is the 1st *vinyasa*. Then, doing *rechaka*, place the hands on the waist; this is the 2nd *vinyasa*. Next, after doing *puraka* and then *rechaka*, place the head slowly on the floor, using the strength of the waist and legs, and do *puraka* and *rechaka* as much as possible; this is the 3rd *vinyasa*. Then, without placing the hands on the floor and doing *puraka*, lift the head up, using only the strength of the waist and legs, and stand up straight; this is the 4th *vinyasa*. Next, after doing *rechaka* and then *puraka*, bring arms out wide at the level of the chest, as described in the 1st *vinyasa*, and hold position; this is the 5th *vinyasa*. (Aspirants should note that in each part of *Prasarita Padottanasana*, both *rechaka* and *puraka* occur in the same *vinyasas*.)

PRASARITA PADOTTANASANA (C)

METHOD

Place hands on waist and stand, doing *puraka*, as in (A) and (B) above; this is the 1st *vinyasa*. Then, doing *rechaka*, lock the fingers behind the back, swell the chest, and stand; this is the 2nd *vinyasa*. Then, doing *puraka* and then *rechaka*, slowly place the head on the floor, straightening and tightening both the arms and legs, and do *puraka* and *rechaka* as much as possible; this is the 3rd *vinyasa*. Then, doing *puraka* and without unlocking the hands, lift the head up, using the strength of the waist only; this is the 4th *vinyasa*. Then, after doing *rechaka* and then *puraka*, unlock the hands from behind the back and place them on the waist; this is the 5th *vinyasa*. Then come into *Samasthiti*.

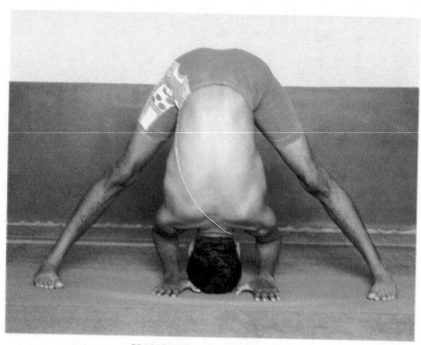

PRASARITA PADOTTANASANA (A)

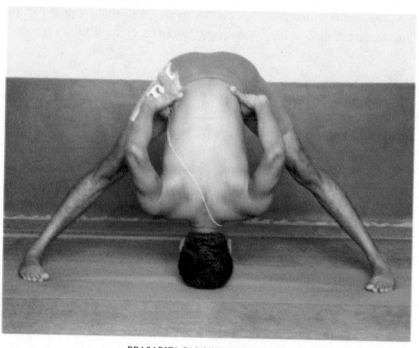

PRASARITA PADOTTANASANA (B)

Prasarita Padottanasana (D)

METHOD

Stand with the legs apart, as in *Prasarita Padottanasana* (A), and doing *puraka*, place the hands on the waist; this is the 1st *vinyasa*. Then, while doing *rechaka*, take hold of the big toes and lift the head, keeping the arms and spine straight; this is the 2nd *vinyasa*. Then, doing *puraka* and again *rechaka*, place the center of the head on the floor in line with the feet, keeping the legs straight and the lower abdomen pulled in, and breathe fully and deeply as much as possible; this is the 3rd *vinyasa*. Next, doing *puraka*, lift the head up completely and hold, doing *rechaka*; this is the 4th *vinyasa*. Then, doing *puraka*, lift the hands, place them on the waist, and return to the position of the 1st *vinyasa*; this is the 5th *vinyasa*. Then follows *Samasthiti*.

BENEFITS

Great attention should be paid to the stomach and the anal channel while practicing the four parts of *Prasarita Padottanasana*. It is best to learn the proper method from a Guru. If this is done, the anal canal will be purified, the bad fat in the lower abdomen will dissolve, the waist will become thin and strong, and the body will become light and beautiful. This *asana* also cures constipation, and purifies the top part of the spinal column and the waist.

6. Parshvottanasana

Parshvottanasana has only five *vinyasas*, the 2nd and 4th of which are the states of the *asana*. *Rechaka* and *puraka* are as in *Trikonasana*.

METHOD

Jump to the right, standing with the legs three feet apart, as described in *Trikonasana*, bring hands together behind the back in a prayer position and, doing *puraka*, turn the right foot and waist to the right, and lift the chest; this is the 1st *vinyasa*. Then, doing *rechaka* slowly, touch the nose to the knee without bending the knees, and hold position, doing *puraka* and *rechaka* as much as possible; this is the 2nd *vinyasa* (*see figure*). Then, doing *puraka*, lift the head up and turn to face the left, following the

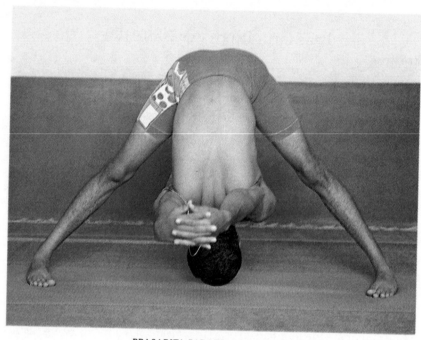

PRASARITA PADOTTANASANA (C)

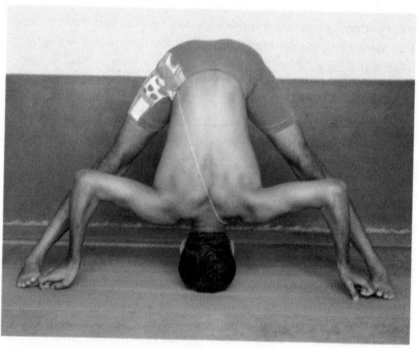

PRASARITA PADOTTANASANA (D)

method for the 1st *vinyasa*; this is the 3rd *vinyasa*. Then, doing *rechaka*, touch the knee with the nose and hold, while doing *puraka* and *rechaka* as much as possible; this is the 4th *vinyasa*. Then, inhale, lift the head and chest, using the strength of the waist, and stand up straight; this is the 5th *vinyasa*. Then, *Samasthiti*.

BENEFITS

Like *Prasarita Padottanasana*, *Parshvottanasana* eliminates the bad fat at the waist, which makes the lower abdomen thin, the waist strong, and the body light.

IN SHORT, ALL THE ASANAS DESCRIBED ABOVE LOOSEN THE LIMBS OF THE BODY, which aids movement and renders the practice of subsequent *asanas* easier. They can be done by men and women of all ages. For people suffering from rheumatic or joint pain, the first and second *Surya Namaskara* and first six *asanas* are especially important. Done properly with *rechaka* and *puraka*, they eliminate the pain that occurs in the joints, and help the body to become light and healthy. It is very important, however, that the particulars of the *vinyasas* above be kept in mind during practice by those who are weak or ill. As these are very difficult to convey to aspirants, however much the correct method for doing the *asanas* is described, it is better that they learn them from a Guru first, and then practice them.

7. Utthita Hasta Padangushtasana

There are fourteen *vinyasas* in this *asana*. The 2nd, 4th, 7th, 9th, 11th, and 14th *vinyasas* are the states of the *asana*.

METHOD

First, join the legs together, hold the arms by the sides, and stand erect. Then, doing *puraka*, place the left hand on the waist, straighten the right arm, raise the right leg, catch hold of the big toe with the right hand, and straighten the knees, chest, and waist (*see figure*); this is the 1st *vinyasa*. Holding this posture and doing *rechaka*, touch the nose to the knee, which is lifted, and hold, doing *puraka* and *rechaka* as much as possible; this is the 2nd *vinyasa*. Then, doing *puraka* slowly, lift the head, straighten the chest

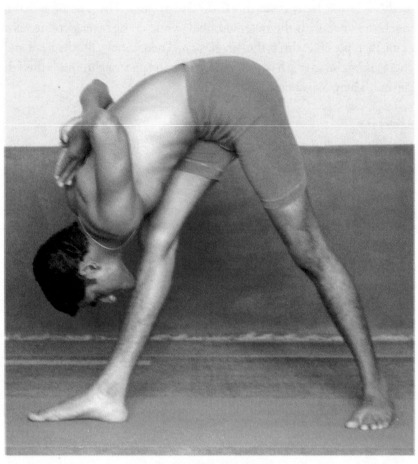

PARSHVOTTANASANA

and waist, and stand as shown in the figure for the 1st *vinyasa*; this is the 3rd *vinyasa*. Next, doing *rechaka*, bring the right leg out to the right, hold the arm, leg, waist, and chest straight, and look to the left, breathing fully and deeply as much as possible; this the 4th *vinyasa*. Then, doing *puraka*, bring the leg back to the center, as in the 1st *vinyasa*; this is the 5th *vinyasa*. Next, doing *rechaka* and keeping the leg lifted, touch the nose to the right knee; this is the 6th *vinyasa*. Then, doing *puraka*, lift the head, straighten the chest and waist, and stand straight, placing the hands on the waist and keeping the raised right leg extended straight, while breathing fully and deeply as much as possible; this is the 7th *vinyasa*. Then, doing *rechaka*, bring the right leg down. Repeat the above for the left leg.

Utthita Hasta Padangushtasana loosens the hip joints, destroys defects of the testicles and male organ of generation, and purifies and strengthens the vertebral column, waist, hips, and lower abdomen. It also eliminates constipation.

8. ARDHA BADDHA PADMOTTANASANA

This *asana* has nine *vinyasas*, the 1st, 2nd, 6th, and 7th of which are the states of the *asana* (*see figure for 2nd* vinyasa). A *sadhaka*, or spiritual aspirant, should practice it under the careful guidance of a Guru.

METHOD

First, stand erect. Then, doing *puraka*, place the right foot on the left thigh, pressing the heel into the lower abdomen, circle the right arm around the back, grasp the right big toe with the right hand, and place the left hand on the waist; this is the 1st *vinyasa*. Next, after doing *rechaka* slowly, bend at the waist, press the left hand to the floor by the side of the left foot, straighten the knee, and touch the knee with nose, doing *puraka* and *rechaka* slowly, as much as possible; this is the 2nd *vinyasa*. Then, doing *puraka*, lift the head only; this is the 3rd *vinyasa*. Next, doing *rechaka* and then *puraka*, stand up straight again, place left hand on waist; this the 4th *vinyasa*. Then, doing *rechaka*, release the right leg, which is in the *Padmasana* form, and straighten it; this is the 5th *vinyasa*. Next, place the left foot on the right thigh, bring the left arm around the back, take hold of the big toe of the left leg with the left hand, as outlined for the right, place right hand on waist, and stand, doing *puraka*; this is the 6th *vinyasa*. Then, as for the 2nd *vinyasa* and doing *rechaka*, bend forward, place the right hand on the floor by the right leg, which is straight, and touch the knee with the nose, doing *puraka* and *rechaka* as much as possible; this is the 7th *vinyasa*. Then, doing *puraka*, lift the head only; this is the 8th *vinyasa*. Next, doing *rechaka* and then *puraka*, place the right hand on the waist and stand up straight; this is the 9th *vinyasa*. (Aspirants should note that *asanas* such as this one which involve both legs are to be performed with the left leg as with the right.)

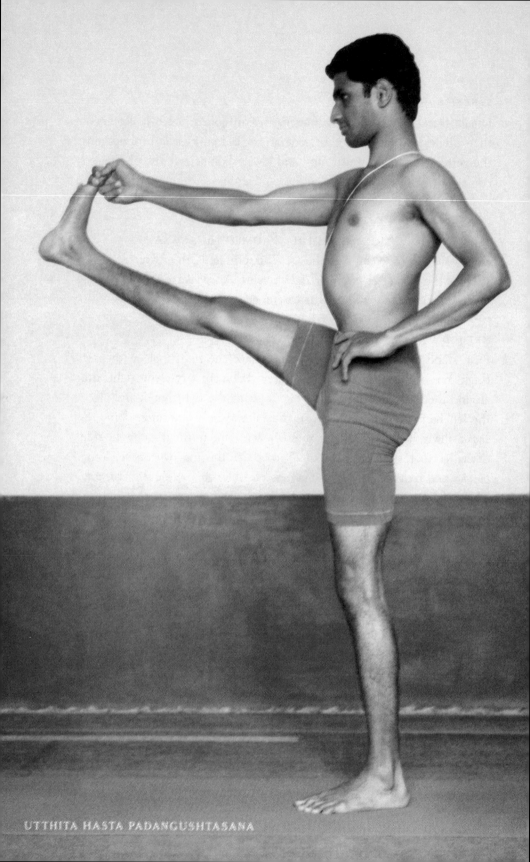

UTTHITA HASTA PADANGUSHTASANA

The rectum, esophagus, and liver are purified by this *asana*. It also pre-vents gas from occurring in the stomach, prevents diarrhea, and quells the gas that arises from inappropriate food. Should gas occur, it wards it off. *Ardha Baddha Padmottanasana* can be practiced by anyone, includ-ing women of all ages, except those whose pregnancies have crossed into the fourth month.

THERE WILL BE DIFFERENCES IN THE STEADINESS OF ASPIRANTS' RECHAKA and *puraka* while practicing the *asanas* described above. If they con-centrate their minds on their breathing only, the state of an *asana* will be spoiled. If, on the other hand, they concentrate only on an *asana*'s state, their *rechaka* and *puraka* will be spoiled. Therefore, it must again be stressed emphatically that these *asanas* be learned under the guidance of an able Guru.

9. Utkatasana

There are thirteen *vinyasas* in *Utkatasana*; the 7th *vinyasa* is its state. The *vinyasa* method described for the first *Surya Namaskara* is important to know for this *asana*.

METHOD

First, begin with the initial six *vinyasas* of the first *Surya Namaskara*. After the 6th *vinyasa* and doing *puraka*, jump into the 1st *vinyasa* of the second *Surya Namaskara*, and perform *rechaka* and *puraka* as much as possible; this is the 7th *vinyasa*. (*Rechaka* and *puraka* for the first six *vinyasas* must be performed in the same manner as in the first *Surya Namaskara*.) Then, doing *rechaka* and *puraka*, press the hands to the floor by the sides of the feet, put the whole weight of the body on the two hands, and lift the body up off the floor; this is the 8th *vinyasa*. Then, doing *rechaka*, throw the body back with the force of the arms, and hold the position, as in the 4th *vinyasa* of the first *Surya Namaskara*; this is the 9th *vinyasa*. Then, doing *puraka*, do the 5th *vinyasa* of the *Surya Namaskara*; this is the 10th *vinyasa*. Next, doing *rechaka*, do the 6th *vinyasa* of the *Surya Namaskara*; this is the 11th *vinyasa*. Then, doing *puraka*, do the 3rd *vinyasa* of the

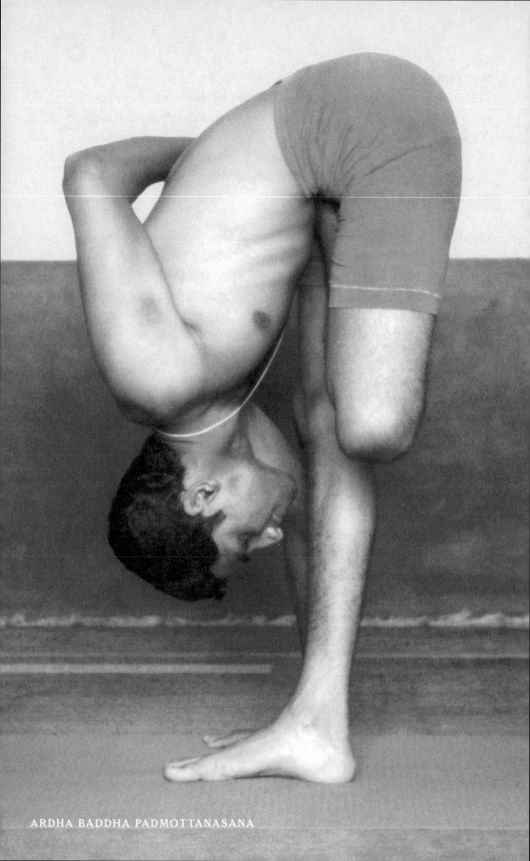

ARDHA BADDHA PADMOTTANASANA

Surya Namaskara; this is the 12th vinyasa. Then, do the 2nd vinyasa of the
Surya Namaskara; this is the 13th vinyasa. Then, Samasthiti.

BENEFITS

Utkatasana increases the strength of the waist, which becomes slender,
and makes the body light. It also prevents pain associated with the vertebral column.

THE VINYASA METHODS FOR THE FIRST NINE ASANAS HAVE NOW BEEN
described. The vinyasas of the asanas that follow begin as they do for
the first six vinyasas of the first Surya Namaskara. Then, from the 7th
vinyasa on, the vinyasas, as well as rechaka and puraka, prescribed for
respective asanas differ. I will try to describe the differences as much as
possible as they occur.

Again, no asana should be performed without following the proper
method of vinyasa. If this is ignored, the organs of the body may not
develop, fat may not be reduced, and the body could grow ill. In addition, some organs may strengthen, while others become weak, or an
organ that was meant to be strengthened may weaken instead. In addition, if there is no steadiness in the movements of rechaka and puraka,
then the balance of the heart could be upset, which could weaken it.
When this occurs, the nadis become spoiled, and when they spoil, all
parts of the body are weakened. Therefore, asanas and the like (puraka,
rechaka, etc.) should be practiced following the methods of vinyasa,
which is best learned from a Guru experienced in yoga shastra. I consider it my earnest duty to caution the reader and aspirant not to try to
learn these methods from books, reflections [photos], or pseudo-yogis.

Hereafter, vinyasa methods are not dealt with deeply. Instead, only
the state of an asana, vinyasa, and their benefits are described. However,
should something special come up, I will describe it.

10. VIRABHADRASANA

There are sixteen vinyasas to this asana, of which the 7th, 8th, 9th, and
10th are the states of the asana. When in the states of Utkatasana and
Virabhadrasana, there is no need to do rechaka and puraka more than five

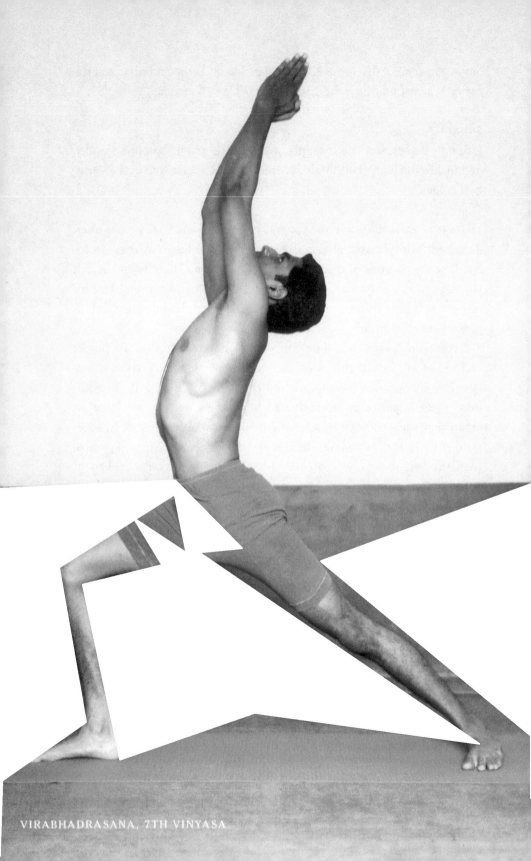

VIRABHADRASANA, 7TH VINYASA

times. However, aspirants should not forget to do *rechaka* and *puraka* while performing the *vinyasas*. In addition, while in the *asana*'s state, it is always important that the body be held firmly and steadily.

METHOD

Begin this *asana* in the same way as the first *Surya Namaskara* and continue through to the end of the 6th *vinyasa*. Next, stand as in the 7th *vinyasa* of the second *Surya Namaskara*, and do *rechaka* and *puraka* five times; this is the 7th *vinyasa* (*see figure*). Then, doing *rechaka*, turn to the left, bend the left knee, keeping the arms raised over the head, with the palms together, the chest lifted up, and do *puraka* and *rechaka* five times; this is the 8th *vinyasa*. Then, keeping the legs in the same position and doing *puraka*, bring arms down to shoulder level, and stand gazing at the fingertips of the left hand, keeping the arms stretched out straight and tight; this is the 9th *vinyasa*. Then, doing *rechaka* and without bending the arms, turn to the right, bend the right knee, and stand gazing at the tips of the right hand with concentration; this is the 10th *vinyasa*. Next, place the hands on the floor on either side of the right foot and, without allowing the legs to touch the floor, lift both the left leg and bent right leg completely off the floor with only the strength of the hands; this is the 11th *vinyasa*. Then, the 12th, 13th, 14th, 15th, and 16th *vinyasas* should be performed in the same manner as the 4th, 5th, 6th, 3rd, and 2nd *vinyasas* of the first *Surya Namaskara*. (*See figures for 9th and 10th* vinyasas.)

Again, it is best to learn the *vinyasas* of all the *asanas*, as well as their states and the series of *rechaka* and *puraka*, under the guidance of a Guru, as these are very difficult to relate in the written descriptions given here.

BENEFITS

By means of *Virabhadrasana*, all the joints of the body, as well as the lower abdomen, spinal column, and organ of generation, are purified. In addition, pain associated with the knees, as well as the pain from standing or sitting all day while working, is eliminated.

11. Paschimattanasana

There are sixteen *vinyasas* to this *asana*. The 9th is its state *(see figures)*.

METHOD

To begin, follow the first *Surya Namaskara* through the 6th *vinyasa*. Then, doing *puraka* and with only the strength of the arms, jump the legs between the hands without allowing them to touch the floor, and stretch out the legs. Then press the hands to the floor on either side of the hips, straighten the chest and waist, lower the head a little, draw the anus up tightly, lift the lower abdomen and hold firmly, and sit erect, slowly doing *rechaka* and *puraka* as much as possible; this constitutes the 7th *vinyasa*. Next, doing *rechaka*, grasp and hold the upper parts of the feet; this is the 8th *vinyasa* (as your practice becomes firm, you should be able to lock your hands behind your feet). Then, doing *puraka* slowly, then *rechaka*, straighten both legs, and place the head between the knees; this is the 9th *vinyasa* and the state of the *asana*. While in the state, do *puraka* and *rechaka* slowly and deeply, as much as possible. Then, slowly doing *puraka*, lift only the head; this is the 10th *vinyasa*. Next, doing *rechaka* and then *puraka*, let go of the feet, press the hands to the floor, bend the legs, and lift the entire body up off the floor merely with the strength of the arms; this is the 11th *vinyasa*. The remaining *vinyasas* are the same as those for the *Surya Namaskara*.

There are three types of *Paschimattanasana*: 1) holding the big toes and touching the nose to the knees; 2) holding on to either side of the feet and touching the nose to the knees; and 3) locking the hand and wrist beyond the feet, and touching the chin to the knee. All three types should be practiced, as each is useful.

BENEFITS

The practice of this *asana* helps the stomach to become slender by dissolving its fat. It also increases *jathara agni* [the fire of hunger], helps food to digest well, and strengthens the organs of the digestive systems (*jirnanga kosha*). In addition, it cures weakness in the hands and legs resulting from a loss of appetite and low digestive fire, as well as indolence and giddiness stemming from an aberration in the liver, and gas problems in the stomach.

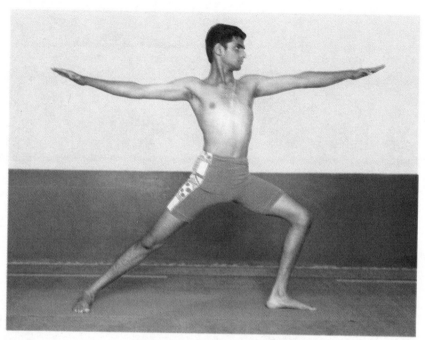

VIRABHADRASANA, 9TH VINYASA

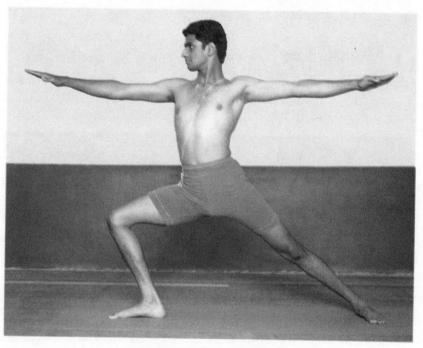

VIRABHADRASANA, 10TH VINYASA

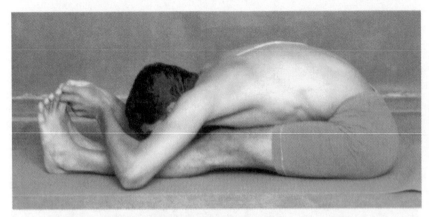

PASCHIMATTANASANA (1st type)

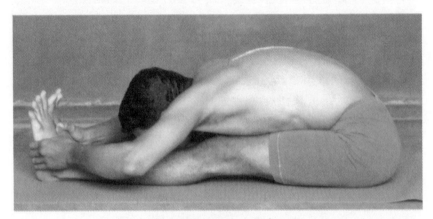

PASCHIMATTANASANA (2nd type)

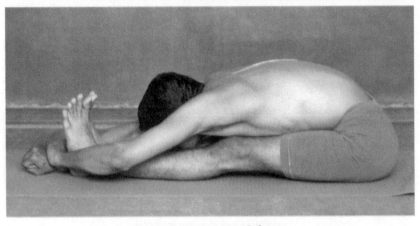

PASCHIMATTANASANA (3rd type)

It is worth noting that, for this *asana*, one has to retract, or squeeze, and hold the anus tightly, as well as squeeze the lower abdomen and hold it in, and concentrate on the *nadis* related to the *kanda*, or egg-shaped nerve plexus in the anal region. As there is no place for the *apana vayu* [downward-flowing *prana*, or energy], which circulates in the anus, to go, it moves upward and becomes one with *prana vayu* [upward-moving *prana*]. When this occurs, an aspirant has nothing to fear from old age and death, as Svatmarama Yogendra, the author of *Gheranda Samhita*, and the sage Vamana both inform us from their own experience:

> *Iti Paschimattanam asanagyam Pavanam*
> *paschimavahinam karoti*
> *Udayam jatharanalasya kuryadudare*
> *karshyamarogatam cha pumsam.*
> [Principle among *asanas*, *Paschimattanasana* causes vital energy to be carried up the spine. As well, it should lead to the rising of the digestive fire, slenderness in the abdomen, and freedom from sickness for all.]
>
> — *Hatha Yoga Pradipika* i : 29

12. PURVATANASANA

Purvatanasana represents *Paschimattanasana*'s opposite. It has fifteen *vinyasas*, of which the 8th is the state of the *asana*.

METHOD

To begin, follow the method for *Paschimattanasana* until the 7th *vinyasa*. Next, place the hands on the floor at a distance of twelve inches behind the waist, lift the legs and torso entirely off the floor doing *puraka*, press the soles of the feet firmly on the floor, lower the head back, making the body firm, and hold, while slowly performing *rechaka* and *puraka*; this is the 8th *vinyasa* (*see figure*). Then, doing *rechaka* slowly, return to the state of the 7th *vinyasa* and sit; this is the 9th *vinyasa*. The *vinyasas* that complete this *asana* follow those of *Paschimattanasana*.

Purvatanasana purifies and strengthens the heart, anus, spinal column, and waist.

ASPIRANTS SHOULD NOTE THAT, IMMEDIATELY FOLLOWING THE PERFORMANCE of an *asana* involving bending the body forward, one that is opposite (that is, one that bends the body backward) is to be done. Similarly, *asanas* in which the body bends backward should immediately be followed by ones bending the body forward. From this, any pain in the waist resulting, for example, from *Paschimattanasana*, will disappear.

13. ARDHA BADDHA PADMA PASCHIMATTANASANA

There are twenty-two *vinyasas* with this *asana*, the 8th and 15th of which constitute its states.

METHOD

To begin, follow the first six *vinyasas* of the first *Surya Namaskara*. Next, sit as in the 7th *vinyasa* of *Paschimattanasana*, stretch the left leg out, place the right leg on the left thigh, pressing the right heel into the navel, bring the right arm behind the back and grasp the big toe of the right foot, take the left foot with the left hand, straighten the head and chest, and do *puraka* slowly; this is the 7th *vinyasa*. Then, doing *rechaka* slowly, place the chin on the outstretched left leg, and do *puraka* and *rechaka* as much as possible; this is the 8th *vinyasa*. Next, doing *puraka* slowly, lift only the head; this constitutes the 9th *vinyasa*. Then, unfolding the legs and crossing them, as in *Paschimattanasana*, lift up the entire body with the strength of the arms; this forms the 10th *vinyasa*. Next come the 11th, 12th, and 13th *vinyasas*, which resemble the 4th, 5th, and 6th *vinyasas* of *Paschimattanasana*. We are now back at the 7th *vinyasa* of the first *Surya Namaskara*. Doing *puraka*, jump the legs through the arms on the strength of the hands alone, stretch the right leg out, place the left leg on the right thigh, grasp the left big toe with the left hand from behind, take the right foot with the right hand, straighten the head and chest; this is the 14th *vinyasa*. Then, doing *rechaka*, place the chin on the right knee, which is stretched out flat, and do *puraka* and *rechaka* slowly, as much as possible;

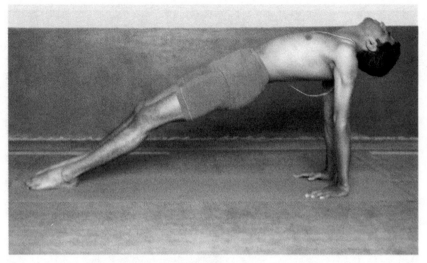

PURVATANASANA

this is the 15th *vinyasa*. Then, doing *puraka*, lift the head only; this forms the 16th *vinyasa*. Next, unfold and cross the legs, lift the entire body up with the hands, doing *puraka*, and stay in this position; this constitutes the 17th *vinyasa*. Then, follow *Paschimattanasana* for the next five *vinyasas* (18th–22nd).

BENEFITS

The practice of this *asana* alleviates the enlargement of the liver and spleen. It also cures abdominal distention due to bad food and activities; the spoiling of the tissues due to a continually provoked *vata*; and weakness due to an inability to take food.[41] Constipation is also cured, and the operation of the bowels is rendered easy.

14. Tiriangmukhaikapada Paschimattanasana

This *asana* has twenty-two *vinyasas*, with the 8th and 15th *vinyasas* constituting its states. The methods of *vinyasa* are the same as those for *Ardha*

---

41 *Vata* is one of the three *doshas*, or functional elements, responsible for each and every activity of the body and provoked by actions and food. When the *doshas* are in harmony, the body is healthy; when they are not, the body becomes ill.

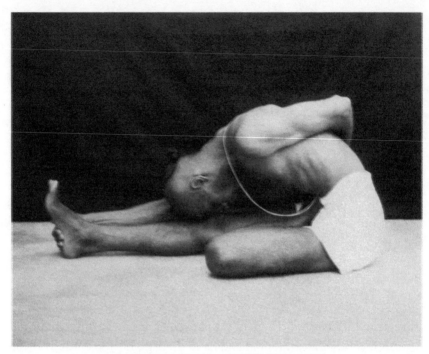

ARDHA BADDHA PADMA PASCHIMATTANASANA

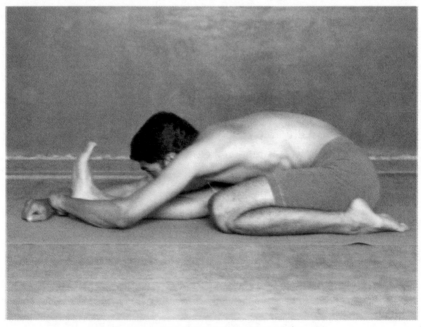

TIRIANGMUKHAIKAPADA PASCHIMATTANASANA

Baddha Padma Paschimattanasana. Indeed, the method of inhaling and exhaling for each *vinyasa* follows the same pattern throughout the *asanas*.

Begin by doing the first six *vinyasas* of the first *Surya Namaskara*. At the 7th *vinyasa*, jump through the arms, sit as described in *Paschimattanasana*, stretch the left leg out, fold the right leg back, placing the right foot by the side of the thigh, join the knees together, take hold with both hands of the left foot, which is at a right angle to the floor, lift the head and chest up fully, and do *puraka*; this constitutes the 7th *vinyasa*. Then, doing *rechaka* slowly, place the forehead on the outstretched leg, and do *puraka* and *rechaka* as much as possible; this is the 8th *vinyasa*. Next, doing *puraka* slowly, lift the head only; this is the 9th *vinyasa*. Then, do the 11th *vinyasa* described in *Paschimattanasana*; this forms the 10th *vinyasa*. The next three *vinyasas*, namely the 11th, 12th, and 13th, follow the 4th, 5th, and 6th *vinyasas* of the first *Surya Namaskara*. Then, while again sitting in the 7th *vinyasa* of *Paschimattanasana*, stretch out the right leg, fold back the left leg in the same manner as the right leg above, take hold of the right foot with both hands, and lift the head and chest up, doing *puraka*; this constitutes the 14th *vinyasa*. Then, doing *rechaka* slowly, place the forehead on the outstretched knee, and do *puraka* and *rechaka* as much as possible; this is the 15th *vinyasa*. Then, doing *puraka* slowly, lift up only the head; this is the 16th *vinyasa*. Next, the 17th *vinyasa* follows the method of the 10th *vinyasa*; the 18th *vinyasa* follows that of the 4th; the 19th follows that of the 5th; the 20th follows that of the 6th; the 21st follows that of the 3rd; and the 22nd *vinyasa* follows the method of the 2nd *vinyasa* of *Paschimattanasana*.

Tiriangmukhaikapada Paschimattanasana cures a number of afflictions, including: body fat; water retention; thighs swollen out of proportion to the size of the body (elephant leg); piles; and sciatica. It also makes the body symmetrical. However, aspirants should not forget to do *rechaka* and *puraka* slowly and as much as possible, while in the state of this *asana*.

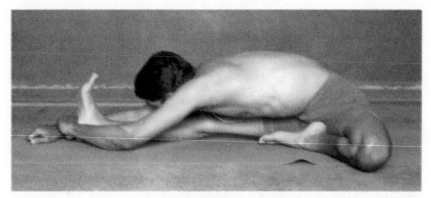

JANU SHIRSHASANA (A)

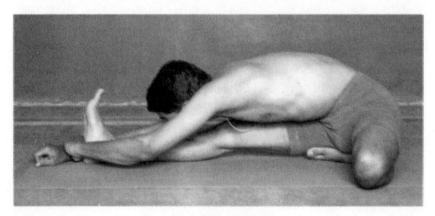

JANU SHIRSHASANA (B)

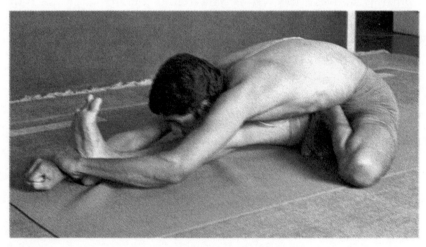

JANU SHIRSHASANA (C)

ASPIRANTS SHOULD NOTE THAT, THROUGH THE 6TH VINYASA OF THE FIRST
Surya Namaskara, the opening *vinyasas* are the same for all the *asanas*. In
addition, all *asanas* conclude with *uth pluthi* [lifting up off the floor with
the strength of the arms], and then a jump back into the 4th *vinyasa* of
the *Surya Namaskara*, followed by the 5th, 6th, 7th, and 8th *vinyasas*.
Aspirants should know the methods for doing these *vinyasas*, as well as for
rechaka and *puraka*. From this point on, I will describe only the *vinyasas*,
the state, and the benefits of an individual *asana*. Readers and aspirants
should learn these fully, which is best done under the guidance of a Guru.
(*To see the state of an* asana, *consult its figure.*)

15. JANU SHIRSHASANA (A)

Janu Shirshasana, which some call *Mahamudra*, is of three types, each of
which has twenty-two *vinyasas*. The 8th and 15th *vinyasas* are their
states. *Janu Shirshasana's* method for *rechaka* and *puraka* follows that of
preceding *asanas*.

FOR ALL THE ASANAS, THE DETAILS OF THEIR BREATHING AND VINYASA
methods, as well as of how to remain in their states in accordance with the
vinyasa method, have to be learned from a Guru. Whatever my descriptions here, there will always be a difference in the actual method of a
practice. For the convenience of the reader and aspirants, however, I have
tried to be as descriptive as possible.

METHOD

For the 7th *vinyasa* of this *asana*, sit as in *Paschimattanasana*, stretch the left
leg out, press the area between the anus and the organ of generation with
the heel of the right foot, pulling the right knee back 90°, bend forward at
the waist, take hold of the foot of the outstretched leg with both hands,
tighten the anus and lower abdomen, straighten the back, lift the head
fully, and do *puraka*. Next, doing *rechaka* slowly, place the forehead or chin
on the knee of the outstretched leg, and do *rechaka* and *puraka* fully as
much as possible; this is the 8th *vinyasa*. Then, doing *puraka*, lift up the
head slowly; this is the 9th *vinyasa*. The next *vinyasas* follow those of preceding *asanas*. This *asana* is to be practiced for both the left and right sides.

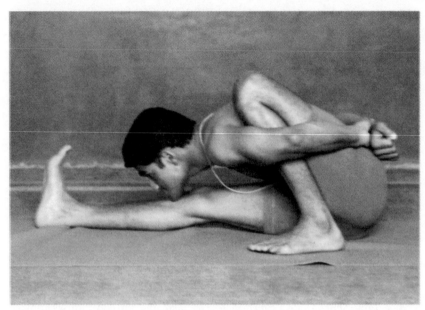

MARICHYASANA (A)

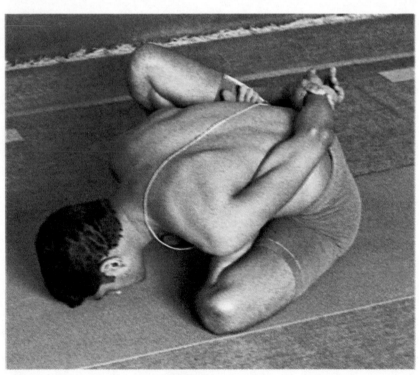

MARICHYASANA (B)

While in the state of *Janu Shirshasana* (A), aspirants should not forget to do *rechaka* and *puraka* as deeply as possible. The reason I repeat this reminder so often is that the bodies of *sadhakas* will become as strong as diamonds through the practice of yoga. They should therefore not allow themselves to become indifferent, but should pursue their practices with faith and reverence.

JANU SHIRSHASANA (B)

METHOD

In the 7th *vinyasa* of this *asana*, sit as in *Paschimattanasana*, stretch the left leg out straight, bend the right knee back 85°, sit the anus directly on top of the right heel, take hold of the left foot with both hands, tighten the anus and lower abdomen, straighten the back, lift the head fully, and do *puraka*. Next, doing *rechaka* slowly, place the forehead or chin on the knee of the outstretched leg, and do *puraka* and *rechaka* as much as possible; this is the 8th *vinyasa*. Then, doing *puraka*, slowly lift the head; this is the 9th *vinyasa*. The next *vinyasas* follow those of preceding *asanas*. The method described above is to be practiced for both the left and right sides.

JANU SHIRSHASANA (C)

METHOD

For the 7th *vinyasa* of this *asana*, again sit as in *Paschimattanasana*, stretch the left leg out straight, bring the right foot in toward the groin, twisting it so that the toes are pressed to the floor and the heel is pointing up toward the navel, press the right knee forward to a 45° angle, take hold of the left foot with both hands, straighten the back and arms, tighten the anus and lower abdomen, and do *puraka*. Then, doing *rechaka* and folding at the waist, place the forehead or chin on the outstretched leg, and press the right heel into the navel, and do *puraka* and *rechaka* as much as possible; this is the 8th *vinyasa* (*see figure*). Again, doing *puraka*, lift the head and straighten the arms; this is the 9th *vinyasa*. The *vinyasas* that follow are as those in earlier *asanas*.

Janu Shirshasana cures maladies such as *muthra krcchra* [burning while urinating], *dhatu krcchra* [semen loss], and diabetes. Fluids secreted by the digestive glands—the pancreas, liver, and so on—break down as a result of poor food habits, excessive coffee drinking, indiscriminate movements, the sight of bad things, poor sleeping habits, excessive sex, intercourse at the wrong times, and eating at the wrong times. When this happens, the liver becomes weak and food fails to digest. The vitality, which results from the transformation of digested food, breaks down and tissues become watery, and a man begins to lose his strength. As he weakens further, his urination becomes difficult to control, and he begins involuntarily to urinate. His organ of generation becomes weak and ailments such as *muthra krcchra* occur. Bedwetting then ensues and his semen is passed out with his urine. Afflictions such as *swapna skalana* [nocturnal emissions while dreaming] soon develop, weakening the body further. If an affliction of this kind overtakes the body, others will quickly follow, bringing death closer. As disorders such as *muthra krcchra* and *dhatu krcchra* are sometimes symptoms of diabetes, it is important to remedy them as early as possible. If one becomes indifferent to them and fails to cure them, then one will develop anemia, which may lead to emaciation and other ailments. It is thus important to be careful regarding these maladies. Medical experts call such ailments *yapya roga*. *Janu Shirshasana* destroys these terrible afflictions, and purifies and strengthens the *nadi* known as *sivani*, which is related to the *dhatu*. As the *sivani nadi* becomes stronger, it destroys defects of the *dhatu*, as well as diabetes. In addition, *Janu Shirshasana* purifies and strenghens the *virya nala*, the *nadi* that connects to the liver and is responsible for creating insulin. *Janu Shirshasana* (A & B) press on the *virya nala* for men, and *Janu Shirshasana* (C) presses on it for women, though all three are necessary and useful for both men and women alike. In this way, diseases of the type just described will be cured, the fire of hunger increased, and food digested easily.

Janu Shirshasana can be practiced by anyone, man or woman—irrespective of age or sex. In this context, I feel duty bound to say that the reason for the overpopulation of today's society is the sensory weakness of our youth. Whenever a person controls his sense organs, he has a limited number of children, produces progeny that are intelligent, healthy, and religious, and lives a long life. Therefore, young men

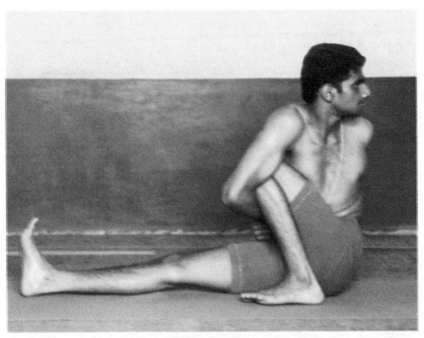

MARICHYASANA (C)

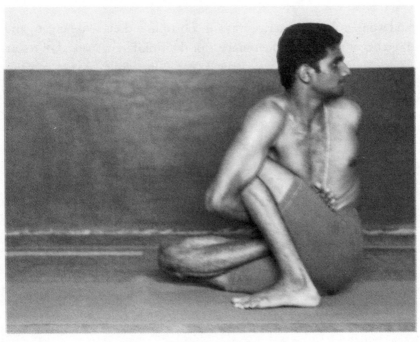

MARICHYASANA (D)

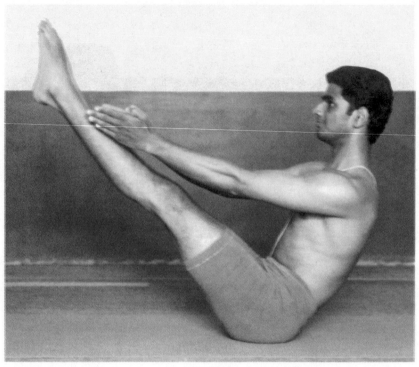

NAVASANA

and women should practice ways of controlling their sense organs and, thereby, of restricting the numbers of their children, instead of resorting to platform speeches or medical operations, which are not very useful.[42] Artificial methods such as these, though helpful to a degree, do not destroy weakness. If our country is to produce robust, intellectual, and long-lived children who believe in God, we must, in my humble opinion, learn ways to control our sense organs. Limiting the number of children is necessary, but it is best to avoid unnatural, allopathic means, which are against nature and bad for the body. Birth control by natural means, on the other hand, helps us to lead long, happy lives, while it, at the same time, nourishes our intellects and frees us from the scourge of disease. Without it, we become subject to sickness, poverty,

---

42 At the time *Yoga Mala* was written, the Indian campaign for population control included "platform speeches" made by government officials who traveled throughout the country in an effort to persuade people about the need for, and benefits of, one-child families.

and shortened lifespans. Aspirants should take this into account. Thus, those that want to lead long, happy lives free from illness, and want to bring forth offspring who are healthy and intellectual, must take to the philosophy of yoga and its practices. This the science of yoga declares like the sounding of a drum. And this I say again to the youth of today, so strongly do I feel about the matter.

By practicing *Janu Shirshasana*, the *dhatu* strengthens and, gradually, the *vasana* of *kama* [the tendency to desire] is destroyed. This is confirmed by the scriptures, and has been my own personal experience as well.

16. MARICHYASANA (A)

There are eight types of *Marichyasana*. The first four are related to yoga *chikitsa* [yoga therapy], and I will describe only these four here. *Marichyasana* was discovered by the sage Maricha, who gave it its name. The first and second forms of the *asana* (A & B) have twenty-two *vinyasas*, and the third and fourth (C & D) have eighteen *vinyasas* each. The states of *Marichyasana* (A) and (B), respectively, are the 8th and 15th *vinyasas*, and of *Marichyasana* (C) and (D), the 7th and 12th *vinyasas*. The methods for the *vinyasas* and for *rechaka* and *puraka* have been specified in earlier *asanas*.

METHOD

To begin, stretch the left leg out as for the 7th *vinyasa* of *Paschimattanasana*, bend the right knee up, pulling the right heel in toward the right buttock, take the right arm around the knee of the bent leg, bring the left hand behind the back and take hold of the right wrist, stretch the left leg, raise the chest, and do *puraka* slowly; this is the 7th *vinyasa*. Then, doing *rechaka* slowly, place the forehead or chin on the knee of the outstretched leg, keeping the outstretched leg straight and tight, and doing *puraka* and *rechaka* as much as possible; this constitutes the 8th *vinyasa* (*see figure*). Next, doing *puraka*, lift the head up; this is the 9th *vinyasa*. Then, *Uth Pluthi* is the 10th *vinyasa*. Practice in this way for both the right and left sides.

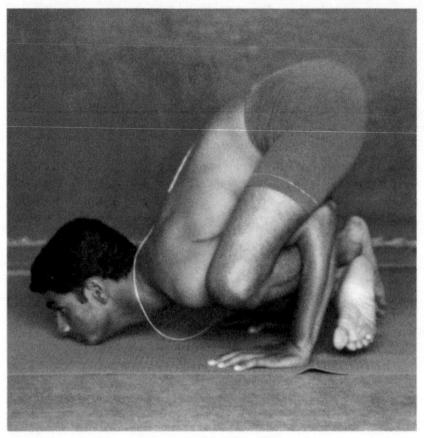

BHUJAPIDASANA, 8TH VINYASA

17. MARICHYASANA (B)

METHOD

Do the first six *vinyasas* of the first *Surya Namaskara*. Then, in the 7th *vinyasa*, sit with the legs stretched out, bring the left heel toward the navel, as in *Padmasana*, bend the right knee, sit firmly with the right knee bent and right heel pulled toward the right buttock, bring the right arm around the right shin, grasp hold of the left wrist with the right hand, and do *puraka*; this is the 7th *vinyasa*. Next, doing *rechaka*, touch the nose to the floor, and do *puraka* and *rechaka* as much as possible; this is the 8th *vinyasa* and the state of the *asana* (*see figure*). Then, doing *puraka*, lift the head and straighten the chest; this is the 9th *vinyasa*. Next, follow the method of *vinyasa* specified in earlier *asanas* and then repeat the above for the left side.

18. Marichyasana (C)

METHOD

First, sit in the same manner as above, stretch the left leg out, press the right foot to the right buttock, as in *Marichyasana* (A), straighten the chest, turn the waist toward the right, bring the left arm around the front of the right knee, twisting the left hand and arm around toward the back, bring the right arm around the back and grasp the left wrist with the right hand, straighten and turn the chest and waist fully, doing *rechaka* and *puraka* as much as possible; this is the 7th *vinyasa*, and the *asana*'s state (*see figure*). The *vinyasas* that follow are specified in earlier *asanas*. In the same manner, practice the above for the left side.

19. Marichyasana (D)

METHOD

Sit, bending the arms and legs as in *Marichyasana* (B), turn the waist, bring the left arm around the front of the right knee and around toward the back, as in *Marichyasana* (C), bring the right arm around the back and take hold of the left wrist with the right hand, turn the waist fully, lift the chest, doing *rechaka* and *puraka* slowly and deeply, as much as possible; this is the 7th *vinyasa* (*see figure*). In the same manner, practice the above for the left leg. The method for the *vinyasas* has been specified earlier.

BENEFITS

The benefits of the four *Marichyasanas* are different, though all cure diseases in accordance with man's physical nature. Aspirants should know this and practice them. They each cure gaseous movements in the stomach and intestines, as well as movements of the rectum, such as diarrhea, and restore digestive power. With that, flatulence, indigestion, and constipation are eliminated. Some women suffer from abdominal pain during menstruation. This is removed by the practice of these *asanas*. The womb becomes powerful and enables a woman to carry a

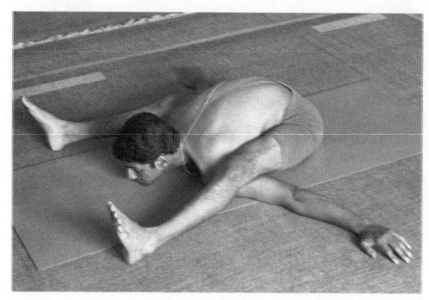

KURMASANA, 7TH VINYASA

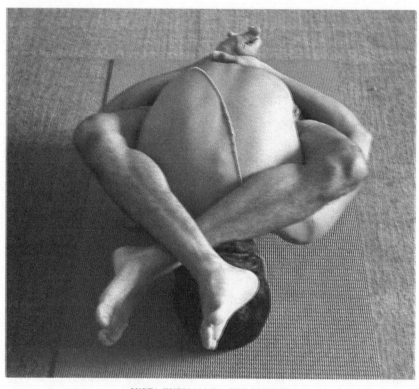

SUPTA KURMASANA, 9TH VINYASA

child strongly, and miscarriage due to weakness is cured. The *vata pitta kosha* [large intestine and gall bladder] are purified, as is the *manipura chakra* [the third chakra at the navel center], and the body gains strength and power. It is a very good idea for women to practice *Marichyasana*, but they should do so under the guidance of a Guru. There should be no error in sitting firmly and holding the hands and legs. Pregnant women should not practice this *asana* after the second month.

20. NAVASANA

There are thirteen *vinyasas* in *Navasana* and the 7th one is the state of the *asana*. The method for the *vinyasas* has been specified earlier.

METHOD

The first six *vinyasas* of this *asana* follow those of the first *Surya Namaskara*. To come into the 7th *vinyasa*, jump the legs in between the arms, doing *puraka* and using only the strength of the arms, and without allowing the body or legs to touch the floor, sit squarely on the buttocks, raise and straighten the legs, sit in the form of a boat, straighten the chest, waist, and legs, hold the arms out straight on either side of the knees, and do *rechaka* and *puraka* as much as possible; this is the 7th *vinyasa* (*see figure*). Then cross the legs without touching the floor, and use the strength of the arms and hands to lift the body up off the floor; this is the 8th *vinyasa*. (While going from the 7th to the 8th *vinyasa*, do *puraka*.) Then, doing *rechaka*, come back to the 7th *vinyasa*. In this way, repeat the *asana* three to six times. The *vinyasas* that follow have been specified earlier. While coming into the state of this *asana*, never do *kumbhaka*, that is, never hold your breath.

BENEFITS

The anal channel, spinal column, ribs, and lower abdomen are purified by *Navasana*. It also cures gastric trouble resulting from food not digesting completely and provoked *vata* due to a lack of digestive fire. The waist additionally gains strength.

21. Bhujapidasana

There are fifteen *vinyasas* in this *asana*, of which the 7th and 8th constitute the states of the *asana*.

METHOD

First, begin with the first six *vinyasas* of the first *Surya Namaskara*. Then, while coming into the 7th *vinyasa* and using the strength of the arms, jump the legs around the shoulders without touching the floor, doing *puraka*, place one foot over the other, squeeze the shoulders forcefully with the thighs, and straighten the arms; this is the 7th *vinyasa*. Then, slowly doing *rechaka* and without touching the legs or feet to the floor, touch only the chin to the floor, and do *puraka* and *rechaka* as much as possible; this is the 8th *vinyasa* (*see figure*). Next, doing *puraka*, come back into the 7th *vinyasa*; this is the 9th *vinyasa*. Then, doing *rechaka*, take back both legs without touching the floor, and balance them on the backs of the arms; this is 10th *vinyasa*. Then, again doing *puraka* and *rechaka*, come into the 4th *vinyasa* of the first *Surya Namaskara*; this is the 11th *vinyasa*. The next *vinyasas* follow those specified earlier.

BENEFITS

Bhujapidasana purifies the *anna nala* [food channel/esophagus], and the body becomes light, and the shoulders and waist become strong.

22. Kurmasana

Kurmasana has sixteen *vinyasas*, the 7th and 9th *vinyasas* of which constitute the states of the *asana*. The state of the 9th *vinyasa* is called *Supta Kurmasana* [Reclined Tortoise] (*see figure*).

METHOD

Begin with the first 6 *vinyasas* of the first *Surya Namaskara*, as specified in earlier *asanas*. In the 7th *vinyasa* and doing *puraka*, jump as in *Bhujapidasana*, lower down to the floor with the strength of the arms, stretch the arms out under the thighs, straighten the legs, put the chin on the floor, lift the head to some extent, and do *rechaka* and *puraka* as much as possible. Then, doing *rechaka*, bring the hands up behind the back and

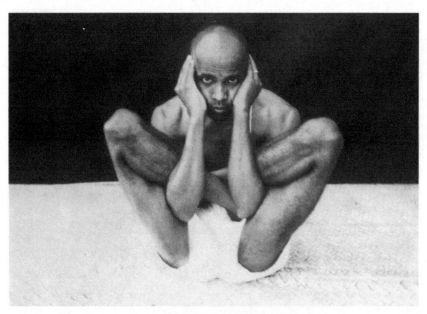

GARBHA PINDASANA

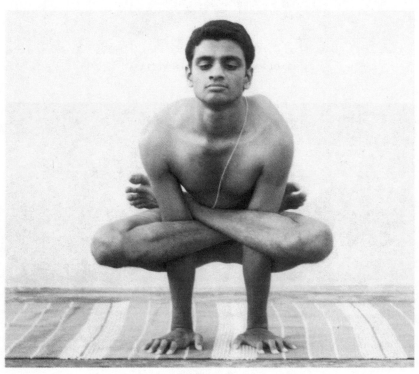

KUKKUTASANA

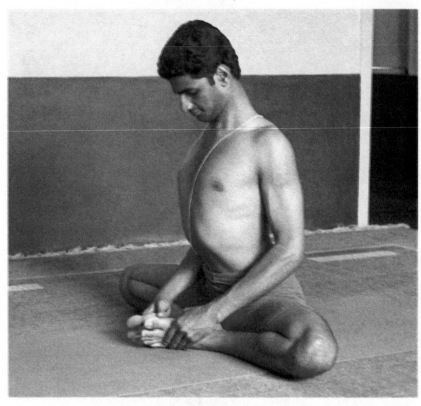

BADDHA KONASANA, 7TH VINYASA

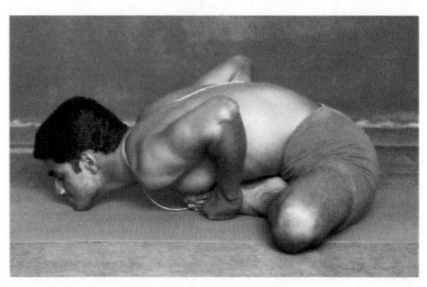

BADDHA KONASANA, 8TH VINYASA

take hold of the wrist; this is the 8th *vinyasa*. Next, cross the legs over each other, put the head on the floor, and do *puraka* and *rechaka* as much as possible; this is the 9th *vinyasa*, the state of which is called *Supta Kurmasana*. The next *vinyasas* follow those of *Bhujapidasana*.

BENEFITS

Kurmasana purifies the *kanda*, or nerve plexus in the anal region from which all 72,000 *nadis* grow. It also purifies the heart and lungs, and eliminates ailments caused by an imbalance of *kapha dosha* [phlegm]. The chest becomes broad, bad fat is dissolved, and the spinal column becomes strong. Chest pain due to over-tiredness is cured, disorders from bad food remedied, and the fat in the lower abdomen dissolved, allowing the body to become healthy.

23. GARBHA PINDASANA

There are fourteen *vinyasas* in *Garbha Pindasana*, the 8th of which is its state *(see figure)*.

METHOD

Begin by doing the six *vinyasas* described in earlier *asanas*, and then sit in the 7th *vinyasa* of *Paschimattanasana*. Next, do *Padmasana* by placing the right foot on the left thigh and the left foot on the right thigh, insert both arms past the elbow through the openings between the thigh and calf, hold the ears with the hands, sitting purely on the buttocks, straighten the chest and spinal column, press both heels on either side of the navel, and remain in this position, doing *rechaka* and *puraka* as long as possible; this is the 7th *vinyasa*. Then, bend the head forward completely, take hold of the head with the hands and, doing *rechaka*, roll back on the spine, keeping the spine rounded. Next, doing *puraka*, roll forward toward the buttocks and, in this way, continue to roll in a clockwise direction until a full circle has been completed, doing *rechaka* on the roll back and *puraka* on the roll forward; this is the 8th *vinyasa*. Next, roll forward and up, pressing the hands to the floor and lifting the body up off the floor, doing *puraka*; this is the 9th *vinyasa*. The *vinyasas* and breathing that follow are described in foregoing *asanas*.

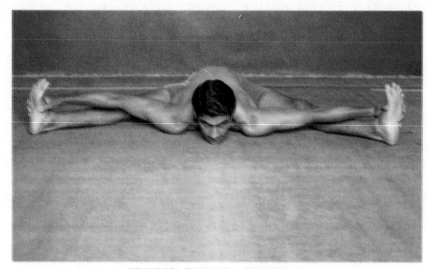

UPAVISHTA KONASANA, 8TH VINYASA

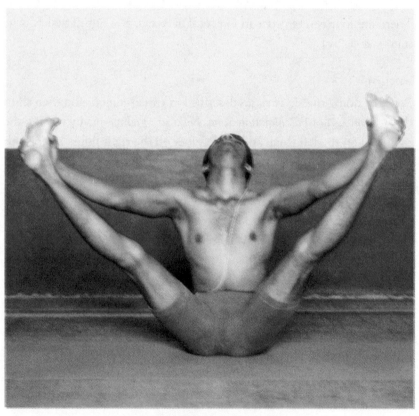

UPAVISHTA KONASANA, 9TH VINYASA

Garbha Pindasana dissolves the fat of the lower abdomen, purifies the manipura, or third, chakra, and wards off diseases of the liver and spleen.

24. KUKKUTASANA

Kukkutasana has fourteen vinyasas, the 8th of which is the state of the asana (see figure).

METHOD

Do Garbha Pindasana above until the 7th vinyasa, which means doing Padmasana and inserting the arms through the space behind the knees. Then, pressing the palms to the floor and doing puraka, lift up the Padmasana, and stand on the strength of the palms; this is the 8th vinyasa. Then, in this position, revolve the stomach (nauli), lift the back and chest fully, and do rechaka and puraka. Next, doing rechaka, come down slowly. The next vinyasas are the same as those for Garbha Pindasana.

When in the state of this asana, one should do rechaka and puraka deeply while keeping the chest, waist, and back completely straight. Then, with the heels pressing on either side of the navel and keeping the head lifted, one should do uddiyana bandha and nauli (see fn. 27). There is no mula bandha in this asana.

BENEFITS

By means of Kukkutasana, the intestines are purified, the fat of the lower abdomen dissolved, and diseases affecting the bowels and urinary tract, as well as excess phlegm, are cured.

25. BADDHA KONASANA

This asana has fifteen vinyasas. The 7th and 8th vinyasas constitute its states (see figures).

METHOD

After doing the first six vinyasas of the earlier asanas, come to the 7th vinyasa of Paschimattanasana, and doing puraka, join the feet, fold them open, press the heels to the *sivani nadi* [the *nadi* between the anus and the genitals], hold the feet open with both the hands, lift the chest, and sit with knees on the floor; this is the 7th *vinyasa*. Next, doing *rechaka*, fold forward, place the head on the floor, and do *puraka* and *rechaka* as much as possible; this is the 8th *vinyasa*. Then, follow the *vinyasas* of earlier *asanas*.

BENEFITS

While in the states of this *asana*, one should do *rechaka* and tighten the anus fully. By pulling the stomach in completely, holding the lower abdomen and anus tightly, and practicing *rechaka* and *puraka*, terrible afflictions related to the anus, such as constipation and piles, will be destroyed, and indigestion will no longer haunt an aspirant. Vamana speaks of *Baddha Konasana* as the greatest of the *asanas*, and says: "*Baddhakonasane tishtan gudamakunchayet buddha gudarognivrittih syat satyam satyam bravimyaham* [The wise one should retract the anus while in *Baddha Konasana* as it wards off anal disease, this I declare is true]." Many have had the experience of being relieved of *bhagandara* [fistula] and *mulavyadhi* [hemorrhoids] by this *asana*. Thus, through its practice, diseases related to the anus and the *dhatu* will definitely be cured.

In this context, a point must be made to readers and aspirants that they should be careful to remember. When one follows the methods of *asana* and *pranayama*, there is no doubt that all diseases will be cured. But if an aspirant thinks that this will occur by his merely practicing *asanas* while continuing to eat *rajasic* [stimulating] and *tamasic* [heavy] foods, then he is misguided. Such a course will actually lead to an increase in sickness.

For diseases related to the anus, *sattvic* and oily foods, such as milk, ghee, half-churned curds, are the best and, of the *sattvic* foods, only those that are thin (*tanu*) should be eaten. Thus, pure and pleasant foods should be consumed. By doing so, someone who is ill, but who practices *asana* and *pranayama*, will become strong in body, mind, sense organs, and intellect, and will be cured. The sick will become free of sickness and the weak will become strong, enabling them to practice subsequent inner steps, such as *pratyahara* [withdrawal of the senses]. However, one should not abandon the practice of yoga after becoming disappointed or indifferent because of an inability to follow the *sattvic* diet strictly. The practice of yoga

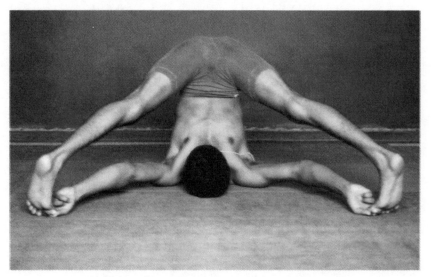

should continue to be pursued while following a diet suited to one's capacity. However, it is good to practice taking *sattvic* foods as much as possible.

26. Upavishta Konasana

Upavishta Konasana has fifteen *vinyasas*, the 8th and 9th of which are the states of the *asana*. The method for the *vinyasas* is described in earlier *asanas*.

METHOD

First, follow the *vinyasas* for the first *Surya Namaskara* through the 6th. Then, doing *puraka* and without touching the floor, jump the legs through the arms purely on the strength of the arms, spread the legs as wide as possible, sit with straightened knees, take hold of the sides of the feet, and lift the head and chest; this forms the 7th *vinyasa*. Then, doing *rechaka*, pull in the stomach, slowly place the head and chest on the floor, and do *puraka* and *rechaka* slowly, as much as possible; this is the 8th *vinyasa*. (As your practice becomes firm, you should be able to rest your chin on the floor in the state of this *asana* while holding your feet.) Next, doing *puraka*, lift only the head, do *rechaka*, and without losing hold of the sides of the feet, come up to sit straight on the buttocks while doing *puraka*, hold the raised legs wide apart and straight, as in the 8th *vinyasa*, keep the chest, arms, and waist straight, look up, and do *rechaka* and *puraka* as much as possible; this is the 9th *vinyasa*. Then, follow earlier *asanas* for the next *vinyasas*.

BENEFITS

While in the states of *Upavishta Konasana*, holding *mula bandha* and *uddiyana bandha* is very important. If the *nadi* called *grdhrasi* [sciatic nerve], which is in the mid-region between the anus and the organ of generation, becomes weak, then the strength of the waist will decrease, and the other *nadis* will weaken as well. When the *grdhrasi nadi* is weak, the waist becomes stiff and sitting and walking become difficult. Through the practice of this *asana*, however, such afflictions will go. With the return of the *grdhrasi nadi's* strength, other *nadis* and organs also will become strong, and *udara bhramana* [gaseous movements in the stomach] will no longer occur, and peristalsis will be resolved. The practice of *Upavishta Konasana*, however, is not appropriate for pregnant women. Otherwise, it is useful for all, men and women alike.

27. SUPTA KONASANA

Supta Konasana has sixteen *vinyasas*. The 8th *vinyasa* is the state of the *asana*.

METHOD

To begin, do the first six *vinyasas* of the first *Surya Namaskara*. Then, doing *puraka*, as in *Paschimattanasana*, lie flat on the floor, legs together, and stretch the legs out tightly; this is the 7th *vinyasa*. Do *rechaka*. Then, doing *puraka*, lift both the legs up and, doing *rechaka*, bring the legs over the head, open them out wide on the floor, and hold the big toes; this is the 8th *vinyasa*. Next, doing *puraka* and without bending the legs, come up into the 9th *vinyasa* of *Upavishta Konasana*, exhale and slowly lower into the 8th *vinyasa* of *Upavishta Konasana*; this constitutes the 9th *vinyasa*. Then, doing *puraka*, lift only the head; this is the 10th *vinyasa*. The next *vinyasas* are the same as those in earlier *asanas*.

The state of *Supta Konasana*, which occurs in the 8th *vinyasa*, comprises lifting the legs, as in *Sarvangasana* [asana 32], doing *rechaka* and

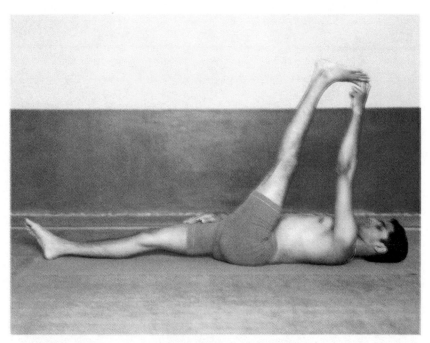

SUPTA PADANGUSHTASANA (1ST PART)

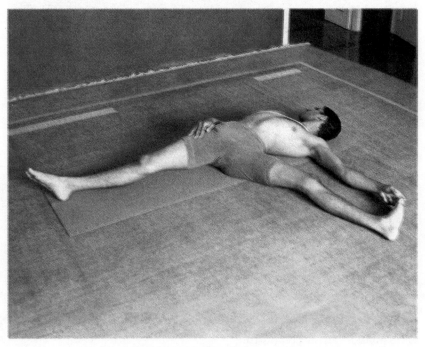

SUPTA PADANGUSHTASANA (2ND PART)

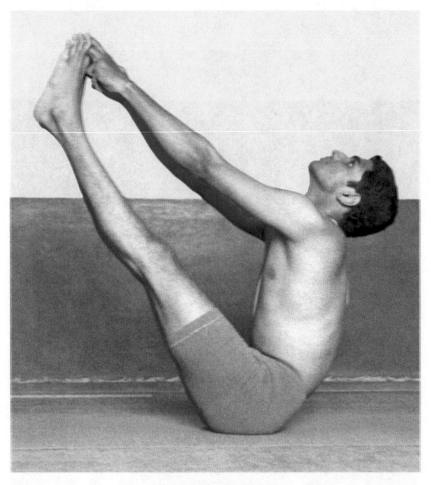

UBHAYA PADANGUSHTASANA

holding the legs as in *Halasana* [*asana* 33], placing the full weight of the body on the shoulders, holding the big toes with the hands, legs wide apart, and doing *rechaka* and *puraka*. While in the state, the abdomen should be drawn in completely, but not with *mula bandha*, or even *uddiyana bandha*. Aspirants should remember this.

BENEFITS
The benefits of *Supta Konasana* are the same as those for *Baddha Konasana* and *Upavishta Konasana*: the *grdhrasi nadi* becomes purified and the spinal column and waist become strong.

28. Supta Padangushtasana

Supta Padangushtasana is a two-part *asana*, the first part consisting of twenty *vinyasas*, and the second of twenty-eight. The 9th and 13th *vinyasas* constitute the states of the first part, and the 11th and 19th *vinyasas*, the states of the second. While in the states of this *asana*, aspirants must be mindful to practice the breathing methods with attention. As this is an *asana* unlike previous ones, I feel prompted to repeat this.

METHOD FOR (PART 1)

First, lie down on the back, as in the preparations for *Sarvangasana* [*asana* 32], doing *rechaka* and *puraka*; this is the 7th *vinyasa*. Then, doing *puraka*, bring the straightened right leg up toward the head, straighten the left leg, strongly take hold of the big toe of the right leg with the right hand, press the left hand firmly on the left thigh, and lie flat, keeping the head on the floor; this is the 8th *vinyasa*. Then, doing *rechaka*, lift only the head a little, touch the nose to the straightened right knee, and do *puraka* and *rechaka* as much as possible; this is the 9th *vinyasa*. Next, doing *puraka*, lower the head to the floor; this is the 10th *vinyasa*. Next, doing *rechaka*, lower the right leg to the floor and join the legs together; this is the 11th *vinyasa*. Repeat the above for the left leg. Then, come into the position of *Halasana* [*asana* 33], press the hands to the floor by the ears, and roll the whole body back over the head, coming into the position of the 4th *vinyasa*. This is called *Chakrasana*. The next *vinyasas* follow those of the previous *asanas*. This is the first part.

METHOD FOR (PART 2)

Perform the first ten *vinyasas* of Part 1. Then, doing *rechaka*, bring the right leg out to the right and lower it to the floor and do *rechaka* and *puraka* as much as possible; this is the 11th *vinyasa*. Then, doing *puraka*, raise the right leg, and return to the 8th *vinyasa* of Part 1; this is the 12th *vinyasa*. Next, doing *rechaka*, touch the nose to the knee; this is the 13th *vinyasa*. Then, doing *puraka*, lower the head to the floor; this is the 14th *vinyasa*. Then, the next *vinyasas* repeat the above for the left side. Indeed, whatever the *asana*, one should practice first on the right side and then on the left side. This is the second part of *Supta Padangushtasana*, both parts of which are very important.

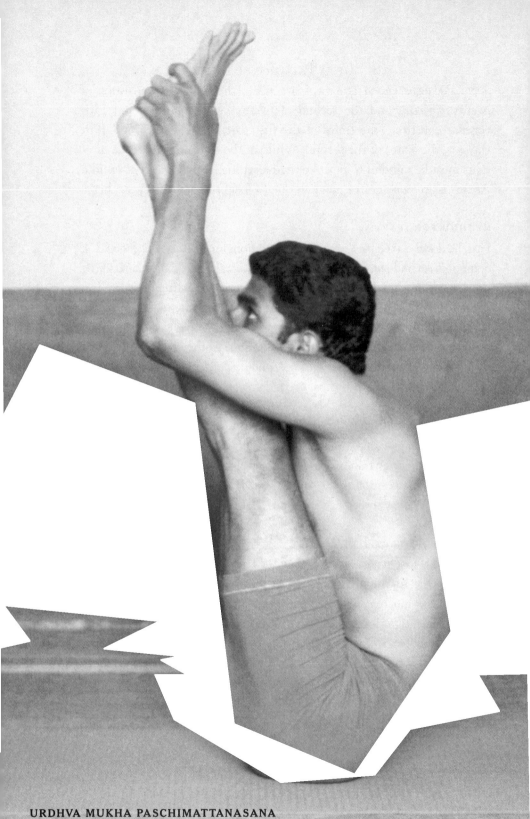

URDHVA MUKHA PASCHIMATTANASANA

Supta Padangushtasana purifies and strengthens the waist region, knees, food and anal channels, and the sperm passageway (*virya nala*). It dissolves the bad fat on the sides of the body and the waist, making the waist slender and strong, and the body light. *Supta Padangushtasana* can be done by all and sundry, except pregnant women.

29. UBHAYA PADANGUSHTASANA

Ubhaya Padangushtasana has fifteen *vinyasas*, the 9th of which is its state.

METHOD

Having reached the 7th *vinyasa* of *Supta Padangushtasana*, lie down and join the legs. Then, doing *puraka*, straighten both legs, as in *Sarvangasana* [*asana* 32], and doing *rechaka*, as in *Halasana* [*asana* 33], bring the legs up over the head, place the feet on the floor, and tightly take hold of the big toes; this is the 8th *vinyasa*. Next, doing *puraka* and without letting go of the toes, roll forward, and come to sit purely on the buttocks in the manner of *Navasana*, doing *rechaka* and *puraka*; this is the 9th *vinyasa*. The next *vinyasas* follow those of earlier *asanas*.

In the 8th *vinyasa* of this *asana*, both *rechaka* and *puraka* occur. Aspirants should note this. While sitting in the 9th *vinyasa*, *rechaka* and *puraka* should be done slowly and as much as possible, and the chest lifted and stomach drawn in fully.

BENEFITS

Ubhaya Padangushtasana is an *asana* that purifies the anus, waist, stomach, genital organs, and the *granthi traya*, or the three knots below the *vina danda*, which begin at the anal canal.[43] It also eliminates the burning sensation that can occur during urination.

---

43 The three knots referred to, known as *Brahma*, *Vishnu*, and *Rudra Granthi*, respectively, are in the subtle body and block the free flow of *prana* from moving up the *sushumna nadi*.

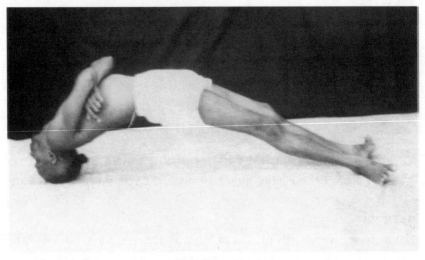

SETU BANDHASANA

30. URDHVA MUKHA PASCHIMATTANASANA

Urdhva Mukha Paschimattanasana has sixteen *vinyasas*, the 10th of which is its state.

METHOD

To begin, lie in the 8th *vinyasa* of *Ubhaya Padangushtasana*, and take hold of the sides of the feet near the heels. Then, doing *puraka*, come into the state of *Ubhaya Padangushtasana* with straightened knees and sitting firmly on the buttocks while holding the feet, not the toes; this constitutes the 9th *vinyasa*. Next, doing *rechaka*, place the face between the knees slowly, then do *puraka* and *rechaka*; this is the 10th *vinyasa* *(see figure)*. Next, doing *puraka* slowly, come back into the 9th *vinyasa* of *Ubhaya Padangushtasana*, and sit. The *vinyasas* that follow are the same as those for *Paschimattanasana*.

BENEFITS

Urdhva Mukha Paschimattanasana purifies the *katti granthi* [lower back], the esophagus, and the *swadishtana chakra*, or region between the anus and navel. When the *swadishtana chakra* is purified, bodily activities become light, all physical activities are free and easy, and impediments, such as disease, do not torture one.

31. Setu Bandhasana

Setu Bandhasana has fifteen *vinyasas*, of which the 9th is the state.

METHOD

Do the first six *vinyasas* specified in earlier *asanas*, and lie down, as in *Supta Padangushtasana*; this is the 7th *vinyasa*. Next, do *puraka*. Then, doing *rechaka*, bend the knees a little, join the heels together, placing the little toes firmly on the floor, bend the head back, place the top of the head on the floor, lift the chest a little, and maintain position, bending the back; this is the 8th *vinyasa*. Then, crossing the arms over the chest and doing *puraka*, lift up the waist and back, and stand straightly on the head and feet alone, while doing *rechaka* and *puraka* as much as possible; this is the 9th *vinyasa*. Then, doing *rechaka* slowly, lie down; this is the 10th *vinyasa*. Next, doing *puraka* again, raise the straightened legs toward the head, press the hands to the floor on either side of the head, do *rechaka*, lift the head and roll the body over on the strength of the arms, and come into the 4th *vinyasa* of the first *Surya Namaskara*; this is the 11th *vinyasa*. The next *vinyasas* follow those of previous *asanas*.

BENEFITS

Setu Bandhasana purifies and strengthens the waist and neck, purifies the *muladhara chakra* [root chakra], and increases the *jathara agni*, or digestive fire. It also purifies the esophagus, heart, and lungs, making them strong.

THE ASANAS DESCRIBED THUS FAR HAVE BEEN ORGANIZED SYSTEMATICALLY AND should only be practiced in the order in which they are presented here, as they purify all the organs of the body in a methodical manner. One *asana* must not be performed at the expense of another, because the muscles on one side of the body will become strong while those on the other will weaken. In other words, the order of these *asanas* should be followed faithfully by aspirants.

Most of the *asanas* just described are related to yoga *chikitsa*, or yoga therapy. Others are *shodhaka* [purificatory]. They can be practiced by anyone, men and women alike, except by women who are more than four months pregnant.[44] Even the very elderly who practice them knowledge-ably will find their bodies becoming soft and light, and increasingly under their own control. This does not mean, however, that they should be learned from pictures or books. On the contrary, they should be practiced under the tutelage of a benevolent *Satguru*. This I repeat over and over again in order that aspirants will remember it.

Following this initial sequence, the succeeding *asanas* can usually be done by one and all. Those described next, especially, should be practiced every day by everyone. Practicing the *asanas* described above every day is also a good idea. When time is short, it is not necessary to practice every *asana*, though those that are done should be practiced in a systematic manner. After a practice becomes firm, it is useful to set aside enough time every day to complete a full practice. Again, the *asanas* I describe next should be practiced daily for good health.

32. SARVANGASANA

Sarvangasana has thirteen *vinyasas*, of which the 8th is its state. As the next five *asanas* are related to *Sarvanagasana*, I will describe their respective fruits collectively.

METHOD

To begin, do the first six *vinyasas* of the first *Surya Namaskara*. Next, coming into the 7th *vinyasa* of *Paschimattanasana*, lie down, arms by the sides and legs straight; this is the 7th *vinyasa*, during which *puraka* and *rechaka* should be done four to five times deeply. Then, with the legs held straight and tightly together, slowly raise the legs up over the head, doing *puraka*, and put the full weight of the body on the shoulders only, hands holding the waist, and elbows pressed to the floor; this is the 8th *vinyasa*. (In the 8th *vinyasa*, the chin should press into the chest properly, the legs be held straight, and the big toes and tip of the nose should form a single line.) (*See figure.*) Stay in this state for five, ten, fifteen, even thirty minutes, doing *rechaka* and *puraka* deeply. Then, lower the legs toward the head, doing *rechaka*, place the

---

44 The *asanas* that should not be practiced by those who are pregnant are *Marichyasana* D and *Garbha Pindasana*.

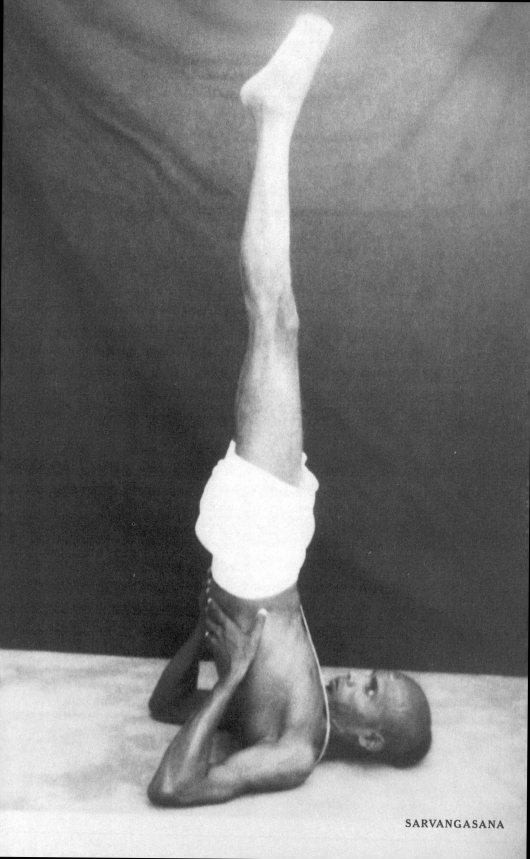

SARVANGASANA

hands on the floor on either side of the head, push the legs back and behind and, lifting the head, come into the 4th *vinyasa* of the first *Surya Namaskara*; this is the 9th *vinyasa*. Then follow the *vinyasas* specified in earlier *asanas*.

33. HALASANA

Halasana has thirteen *vinyasas*, the 8th of which is the state of the *asana*.

METHOD

Do the first seven *vinyasas* described in *Sarvangasana*. Then, doing *puraka*, join together and raise the legs, as in *Sarvangasana*, and doing *rechaka* slowly, lower the legs to the floor over the head, keeping them straight, place the feet on the floor, lock the fingers behind the back, arms tight and straight, press the chin into the chest without bending the legs, and do *puraka* and *rechaka* deeply, as much as possible; this constitutes the 8th *vinyasa*. The next *vinyasas* follow those of *Sarvangasana*. Aspirants should note that *rechaka* and *puraka* both occur in the 8th *vinyasa*.

34. KARNAPIDASANA

There are thirteen *vinyasas* in this *asana* and the 8th is the state of the *asana*.

METHOD

To start, lie down, as in *Sarvangasana*; this is the 7th *vinyasa*. Then, doing *puraka*, proceed to the 8th *vinyasa* of *Sarvangasana*, which is *Karnapidasana*'s state and, doing *rechaka*, lower the legs to the floor, as in *Halasana*, bring the knees to the floor, take hold of the ears tightly with the knees, lower the arms to the floor, lock the fingers, and do *puraka* and *rechaka* as much as possible; this is the 8th *vinyasa*. In the state of this *asana*, the stomach should be drawn in fully without tightening the anus, and *rechaka* and *puraka* performed.

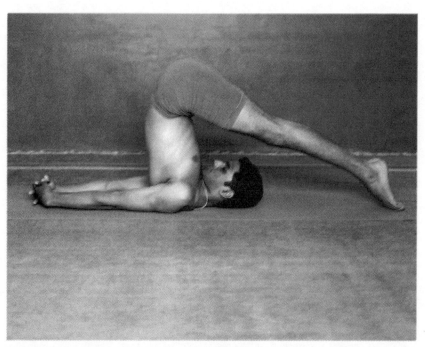

HALASANA

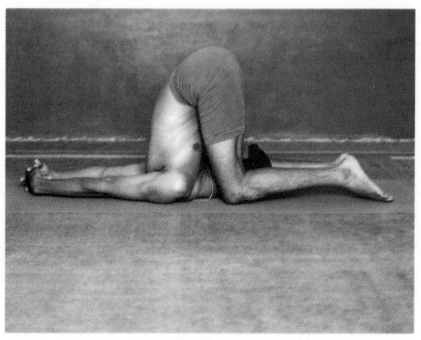

KARNAPIDASANA

35. Urdhva Padmasana

Urdhva Padmasana has fourteen *vinyasas*, of which the 9th *vinyasa* is its state.

METHOD

Do all *vinyasas* outlined above through to the state of *Sarvangasana*; this is the 8th *vinyasa*. Then, maintaining the same state and doing *rechaka*, do *Padmasana*; this is the 9th *vinyasa*. While in this state, tighten the anus, draw in the stomach fully, hold the knees with the hands, straighten the arms, and slowly do *puraka* and *rechaka* as much as possible. Then, doing *puraka* and *rechaka*, unlock the legs and come into the 4th *vinyasa* of *Sarvangasana*; this is the 10th *vinyasa*. The subsequent *vinyasas* are as those for *Sarvangasana*.

36. Pindasana

Pindasana has fourteen *vinyasas*. The 9th is the state of the *asana*.

METHOD

First, follow the *vinyasas* of *Urdhva Padmasana* above through to the 9th *vinyasa*; this is the 8th *vinyasa*. Then, doing *puraka* and then *rechaka*, bring the legs in *Padmasana* slowly down to the forehead, envelop the thighs with the arms, embrace the *Padmasana*, hold the wrists tightly, balance the body on the shoulders only, and slowly do *puraka* and *rechaka* as much as possible; this is the 9th *vinyasa*. Subsequent *vinyasas* are as those of *Sarvangasana* (*see figure*).

MOST PEOPLE WITH SOME KNOWLEDGE OF YOGA KNOW ABOUT SARVANGASANA. They may not know the method for the *vinyasas*, but it is my belief that they have heard, at least, of *Sarvangasana* itself. What they may not be aware of, however, is the order in which the *asanas* associated with it must be performed, or how steady to make the *rechaka* and *puraka*, or how much time to devote to their practice. This is because they get their information from books on the practice of yoga written by people who want to spread word of the science of yoga out of a love and respect for it, but without knowing it properly themselves. If we read these books, we notice

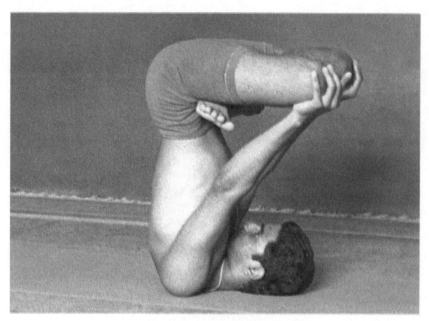

URDHVA PADMASANA

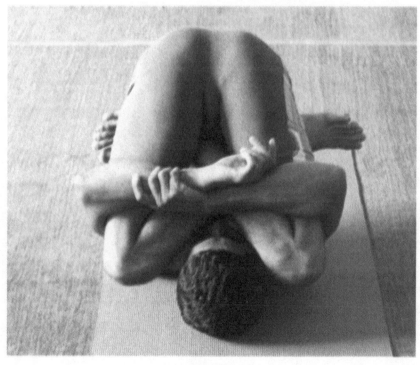

PINDASANA

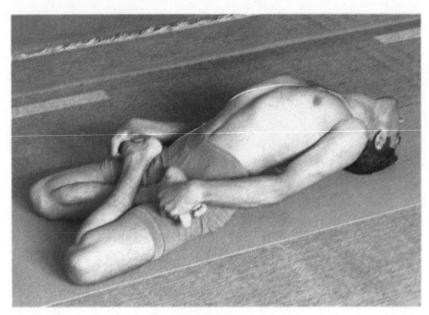

MATSYASANA

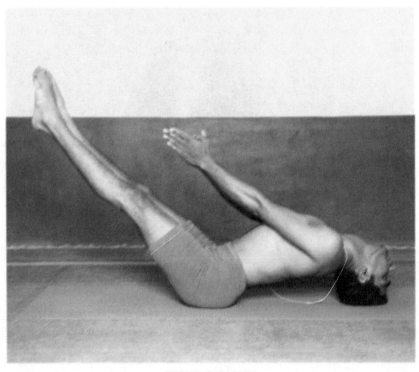

UTTANA PADASANA

that the relation between one *asana* and another, and a description of *rechaka* and *puraka*, are nowhere to be found; moreover, in such books, differences regarding the methods of practice abound.

It is my view that it is better to put accurate knowledge before aspirants. I have thus tried to write this book in such a way that, if readers follow its methods properly, they will derive some benefit from what it describes. In the modern world, people have many kinds of fears and inaccurate notions about the science of yoga. In order to allay such fears and correct such notions, the path of yoga should first be practiced in accordance with the scriptures, its fruits experienced, and then be passed on to others. As many great people in the world are knowledgeable about the science of yoga, they should foster able disciples, direct them on the proper path, and then send them forth for the benefit of the universe. It is not enough to lecture: "Simply do it; you will profit." One must be able to demonstrate what one speaks of. This is the prime goal of yoga.

The *shastrakaras* refer to *Sarvangasana* and *Shirshasana* [*asana* 39] as "*viparita karani*."[45] Just as a country's king and ministers are important, so too, for the practice of *yoganga* [yogic limbs], are these two *asanas* important. Accordingly, having started with the *Surya Namaskara* and then proceeded through all the other *asanas*, one should end with these seven *asanas*, the order of which must never vary: *Sarvangasana*; *Halasana*; *Karnapidasana*; *Urdhva Padmasana*; *Pindasana*; *Matsyasana*; and *Uttana Padasana*.

Again, these seven *asanas* must be practiced systematically; after finishing them, one should never go on to do an *asana* like *Paschimattanasana*. Only the five *asanas* just described and those ahead— *Matsyasana*, *Uttana Padasana*, and *Shirshasana*—should be practiced after all the other *asanas* have been done. Otherwise, it could be harmful to an aspirant. Therefore, one should practice following only the methods specified here. This is the rule, which must never be forgotten.

BENEFITS OF ASANAS 32 TO 36

Some of the five *asanas* just described strengthen the skeletal muscles, others purify different parts of the body, and still others purify and

---

45 "*Viparita karani*" means inverted, turned around, or working in a contrary manner, and refers to the shoulder stand and headstand.

strengthen the inner *nadis, chakras, sira, dhamani* [blood vessels and neural network], three *doshas*, digestive system, and the *jathara agni*.

Normally, the food we eat mixes with bile and is well digested, with the result that the essence of the digested food becomes blood. The transformation of every thirty-second drop of blood is vitality, and the thirty-second transformation of this vitality is called *bindu* [nectar; droplet], which is also known to yogis as *amrita bindu*, or drop of immortality. *Amrita bindu* pervades all parts and limbs of the body, strengthening, nourishing, and soothing them. As long as *amrita bindu* remains in the body, life abides in the body. But when *amrita bindu* attenuates, death is drawn closer. As a scriptural statement states: "*Maranam bindu patena jivanam bindu dharanat* [The falling of the drop is death, while retaining *bindu* is life]." Therefore, we have first to preserve *amrita bindu*. It has to be purified and preserved properly, and this can be achieved by no other method than *Sarvangasana* and the other *asanas* outlined above. These five *asanas* purify all parts of the body, and stimulate *bindu* to pervade it. *Sarvangasana* purifies the heart, lungs, and all other parts of the body by making the blood hot. That is probably why it has earned the name *Sarvangasana*.[46]

By means of these five *asanas*, the *vishuddhi chakra* [throat chakra], heart, lungs, limbs, digestive system, and *jathara* [stomach] are purified, and perversions of the vital wind, which result in hiccups, dry cough, constipation, and indigestion, as well as high blood pressure, are warded off. They also prevent illnesses such as asthma, and ailments related to the heart. Doctors believe that changes in the *vata, pitta,* or *kapha dosas* cause disease. If there is a change in the *kapha dosa*, the defective *kapha* increases and travels to the lungs, where it congeals and impedes respiration, weakening the body. Such a disease results from contact with contaminated food, *vihara dosa* [inappropriate recreation], or contact with contagious people.

Illnesses related to the heart and *nadis*, doctors believe, are *yapya*, or congenital; they are a deformation of *prakriti* [nature]. Medical cures for *yapya rogas* are futile; though the treatments for them may lead a person to feel better for a while, they can never be fully successful. Like a thorn in a leg that is removed by another thorn, these diseases are not curable by medicine. Allopathic doctors are unable to cure them and, after look-

---

46 *Sarvangasana* [*sarva-* all + *anga-* limbs + *asana-* pose]

ing into the yoga *shastras*, they have rightly begun to believe that many physical and mental ailments can be remedied by natural therapies, which is the path of yoga.

Sarvangasana cures all diseases, purifies the *vishuddhi chakra*, and makes the *amrita bindu* firm. *Halasana* purifies the intestines, the region of the waist, and the throat channel, and strengthens them. By means of an *asana* such as *Sarvangasana*, ailments of the throat or those likely to affect the throat, are destroyed, including the inability to pronounce words clearly, throat pain, and diseases associated with the heart. *Sarvangasana* also purifies the base of the throat (*kanta kupa*), prevents choking, and stops the appearance of boils caused by internal heat. In addition, musicians who practice this *asana* for a period of time will find that it helps their singing become melodious and tuneful.

Karnapidasana eliminates diseases of the ears, such as those that cause pus and blood to flow frequently, or a ringing in the ears. If such things are ignored, men gradually lose their hearing. It is thus better to cure them as early as possible with *Karnapidasana*.

Urdhva Padmasana purifies the anal and urinary channels, and causes the anterior section of the spinal column to become firm.

Pindasana purifies the lower abdomen, the spinal column, liver and spleen, and the stomach.

The five *asanas* associated with *Sarvangasana* involve bending the body forward. The next two, namely *Matsyasana* and *Uttana Padasana*, bend the body back.

The five *asanas* described above must be practiced systematically. After practicing them, an aspirant should not go on to practice other *asanas*, such as *Paschimattanasana*. Following these five, *Matsyasana*, *Uttana Padasana*, and *Shirshasana* should be practiced. To do otherwise would be harmful to an aspirant. Therefore, the method specified here should be followed during practice. This is the *niyama* [rule], which an aspirant should never forget.

37. MATSYASANA

Matsyasana has thirteen *vinyasas*, the 8th of which is its state.

To begin, lie down, as in *Sarvangasana*; this is the 7th *vinyasa*. Then, doing *puraka* and *Padmasana*, press the hands to the floor on either side of the head and, doing *rechaka*, lift the head up and place the crown of the head on the floor, bend the back up by lifting the waist, take hold of the feet, straighten the arms, and do *puraka* and *rechaka* as much as possible; this is the 8th *vinyasa*. Then, do *puraka* and next *rechaka*, lower the head, unfold the legs from *Padmasana*, hold the legs and feet as in *Halasana*, place the hands next to the ears and roll over into the 4th *vinyasa* of the first *Surya Namaskara*; this is the 9th *vinyasa*, which is called *Chakrasana*. The next *vinyasas* are the same as those in earlier *asanas*.

38. UTTANA PADASANA

Uttana Padasana has thirteen *vinyasas*, of which the 8th is its state.

METHOD

Perform all the *vinyasas* from the beginning of *Sarvangasana* to the 7th *vinyasa*; this is also the 7th *vinyasa* of *Uttana Padasana*. Then, as in *Matsyasana* above, lift the head, place the crown of the head on the floor, arch the back, extend the legs, as in *Navasana*, hold straightened arms out parallel with the legs, bring the palms together, tighten the entire body, and do *rechaka* and *puraka* as much as possible; this is the 8th *vinyasa*. Then do the 9th *vinyasa* of *Matsyasana*, and roll into the 4th *vinyasa* of the first *Surya Namaskara*; this is the 9th *vinyasa*. The next *vinyasas* follow those of earlier *asanas*.

BENEFITS OF ASANAS 37 & 38

Matsyasana and *Uttana Padasana* counterpose the five *asanas* that precede them and remove the shoulder and waist pain that result from their practice. They also purify the esophagus and anus, as well as the liver and spleen, and furnish the waist and neck with increasing strength. *Matsyasana* and *Uttana Padasana* should be practiced after *Sarvangasana* and the like are completed.

I HAVE DESCRIBED EACH OF THE SEVEN ASANAS ABOVE AND THEIR VINYASA methods separately to help aspirants better understand them. However, it

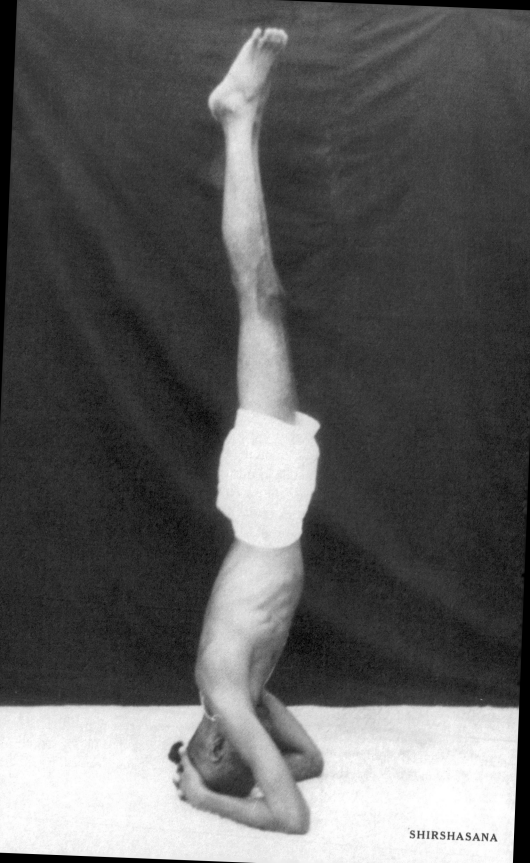

SHIRSHASANA

is not necessary to do all the *vinyasas* specified for each *asana*, as this would take a very long time. Instead, one should practice consolidating them, after having clearly grasped the importance of the steadiness of *rechaka* and *puraka*. Thus, after *Sarvangasana*, one should do *Halasana*, then come into the state of *Karna Pidasana*, followed by *Urdhva Padmasana*, then do *Pindasana* and, finishing *puraka*, move into the state of *Matsyasana* while doing *rechaka*, and then, pass into the state of *Uttana Padasana*, and finally, doing *puraka* and *rechaka*, do *Chakrasana*. Aspirants should keep this method in mind.

39. SHIRSHASANA

Some people call this *asana Kapalasana* or *Viparita Karani* but, as it is most commonly known as *Shirshasana*, we have called it so as well. *Shirshasana* has thirteen *vinyasas*; the 8th constitutes its state. (Pregnant women should not practice this *asana*.)

METHOD

While coming from the 6th to the 7th *vinyasa* of the first *Surya Namaskara* and doing *puraka*, sit on the knees, lock the fingers together and place the elbows on the floor; this is the 7th *vinyasa*. Then, doing *rechaka* and then *puraka*, place the crown of the head on the floor, interlocked hands cupping the back of the head and, doing *rechaka* and *puraka* again, straighten the legs and, keeping them together and straight, lift them up with the power of the arms, tighten the body, point the toes, and keep the body erect using the strength of the arms; this is the 8th *vinyasa*, during which *rechaka* and *puraka* should be done slowly and as many times as possible. Then, doing *rechaka* slowly, bring the feet back down onto the floor, rest with the buttocks on the heels and the head on the floor for two minutes. Next, doing *puraka* and then *rechaka*, jump back into the 4th *vinyasa* of the first *Surya Namaskara*; this is the 9th *vinyasa*. The next *vinyasas* are as those described above.

Aspirants should note that merely putting the head down and legs up, and then standing upside down is not *Shirshasana*; very simply, this is wrong. Indeed, no one should be deluded into thinking that *Shirshasana* is an easy *asana*. The proper method for it must be carefully learned. For

BADDHA PADMASANA

example, *the entire body must stand upside down on the strength of the arms alone.* If the full bodily burden is carried by the head, the circulation of the blood from the heart, which is flowing properly to the limbs, will be prevented from making its way to the subtle *nadis* in the crown of the head, which is pressed to the floor. Then, following the descent from the state of the *asana*, there is the possibility that the subtle *nadis* in the brain could become spoiled by the inrush of blood when the head is lifted. This could impede bodily and intellectual growth, and lead to delusions, mental abnormalities, illness, or a shortened life. Aspirants should therefore practice this *asana* knowledgeably and with great care. Some people, ignorant of the proper method, practice *Shirshasana* after seeing it in a book or photograph, and so subject themselves to numerous problems, and even inspire fear in others who practice the *asana* correctly, as I have witnessed from my own experience. I have also come across situations in which many ailments resulting from the improper practice of this *asana* have been cured by an aspirant's learning the method properly. Thus, let me repeat again that aspirants should take great care with *Shirshasana*.

Some say that practitioners should stay in this *asana* for only two to five minutes; otherwise, harm could come to them. It must be stressed, however, that this is not correct, as the following scriptural saying attests: "*Yama matram vashe nityam* [We can dwell in (*Shirshasana*) for three hours]." This is a view supported by experienced and learned people well-versed in the scriptures. It is also the right one. One *yama* equals three hours. To be able to stay in *Shirshasana* for three hours, an aspirant should begin by practicing it first for five, then ten, and then fifteen minutes, that is, he should gradually increase the time in the state of *Shirshasana* by increments of five minutes. In this way and by force of slowly practicing over many days, months, and years, an aspirant should be able to stay in the *asana* for a full three hours. Practiced in this way, *Shirshasana* will nourish the body, sense organs, mind, and intellect, and thereby promote their evolution. However, if an aspirant stays in the state of *Shirshasana* for one to five minutes, or even less than a minute, he will not get the specified benefits.

In *Shirshasana*'s state, both the lower abdomen and the anus should be taken in fully and held tightly—in other words, *mula bandha* should be done. In addition, the entire body should be kept erect and *rechaka* and *puraka* performed deeply, without *kumbhaka*.

Through the practice of *Shirshasana*, the subtle *nadis* of the head—that is, those related to the brain and sense organs, such as the eyes—are purified by an inflow of warm blood, and the power of memory is increased. Eye disease is destroyed, the eyes glow, and long-sightedness improves. The five sense organs, too, become purified. Moreover—and by means of this *asana* only—the *bindu* that results from the transformation of food into blood and is preserved through pure food and fresh air (both of which are needed for the body's survival) is able to reach the *sahasrara chakra* (the seventh and highest chakra, where spiritual illumination occurs). Knowledgeable people regard the attenuation of *amrita bindu* as death and its preservation as life. It is better, therefore, to preserve it. As long as there is pure *bindu* in our bodies, fresh youthfulness will be manifest in us. As experience demonstrates again and again, practicing without fail for a long time not only endows the body with power and brightness, but increases intellectual power. This is affirmed by the yoga *shastra*: "*Maranam bindu patena / Jivanam bindu dharanat / Tasmat sarvaprayatnena / Bindu dharanam abhyaset* [Loss of *bindu* is death / and the preservation of it, life / So, by all means / is the holding of *bindu* to be preserved]."

To repeat, with *bindu*'s loss comes death; with its retention, life. Thus men should practice to preserve it with all their might. And preserving *bindu* is what *Shirshasana* does. Yet no amount of writing can convey the utility of this *asana*. An aspirant can only enjoy its happiness through its practice. It is impossible to try to describe the sweetness of sugar. Only by tasting sugar can the experience of its sweetness be had, even for Brahma [God]. Just as people feel the sweetness of sugar by eating it, so too will they experience the happiness of this *asana* by practicing it.

As I mentioned earlier, there are differences of opinion about the practice of *Shirshasana* and other *yogasanas*. According to some, delusions and other afflictions result from the over-practice of *Shirshasana*, and it may also weaken the heart. Indeed, it is claimed that it is harmful to practice for any amount of time. This, at least, is the theory propounded in books written by publicity-hungry people who may or may not practice yoga, or who call themselves yogis out of some attachment to the yogic science. And, to some extent, their words are true, at least for those who think they are practicing *Shirshasana* when they put their heads down on

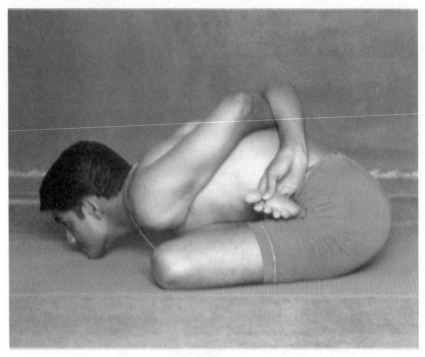

YOGA MUDRA, BADDHA PADMASANA, 9TH VINYASA

the floor and their legs up in the air whenever the fancy strikes them. Not surprisingly, such theories create great fear in people who have the zeal, godly devotion, and desire to practice yoga, and those that advance them gain names for themselves and great fame. After all, when someone achieves something others have not, can fame not come as a result? But there are no grounds for such wrongheaded notions whatsoever. Indeed, if there were any danger in yoga, people long ago would have lost interest in the science, become indifferent to its practice, and declared its sayings, the sayings of the greatest of the great yogis, such as Patanjali, to be a bundle of myths.

But how can there be any danger if one follows the path of those who have studied the *shastras* fully, correctly, and in the traditional manner, and who understand their meaning; where can be the harm if one reads the scriptures properly, understands them rightly, and practices under the guidance of a pious Guru for many years, and gains experience, and follows the path of people of this kind? For the great souls of the world who, toiling incessantly, have renounced all pleasures and wealth, thinking that selfless service is man's true goal, and who, knowing yoga's real nature first themselves, have resolved to help others, seek nothing else in the world but this service. Thus, as these great souls are the helpers of the world, then to follow their path and learn the scriptures correctly is to find no danger come to oneself.

Claims are also made that *Shirshasana* or yoga of any kind should not be practiced by people after they have reached the age of forty. This is not borne out by experience or by the *shastrakaras*. After all, great seers such as Patanjali brought us the science of yoga for the cure of diseases and, very naturally, embodied beings are prone to things of this kind. Do diseases not haunt men after forty?

The body is the abode of disease. If it is tired due to a lack of food, sleep, or the like, or from great difficulty or poverty, disease will overtake it. Therefore, it is essential to cure it of its ailments. From this standpoint, as the mind weakens in old age, the sense organs weaken, too. When the mind is weak, diseases can easily overtake the body. Therefore, a mental cure too is a must. In short, there is no age restriction for the practice of yoga. As the *shastrakaras* say: *"Yuva vrddho'tivrddho va vyadito durbalo'pi va / Abhyasat siddhim apnoti / Sarvayogeshvatandritah* [Whether young or old, or very old / sick or debilitated / one who is vigilant attains, by means of practice, success in all the yogas.]"[47] This means that whether one is young or old ("old" here meaning above sixty years of age, and "very old," beyond ninety), whether one is a woman or a man, or suffering from a disease or weakness, if one practices yoga, then one can attain perfection. Indeed, anyone—men and women of all ages, sick or weak—can practice yoga, except those who are lazy.

Finally, it is the claim of some books that *Shirshasana* should be the first *asana* aspirants practice, followed by the others. This is contrary to the scriptures and not borne out by experience. Moreover, such a claim is made by those who do not know the nature of the body. *Shirshasana* always creates peace of mind and alleviates the fatigue of the body. According to experts in the field of the *Ayurveda shastra*, as well as those experienced in the subject, if one does *Shirshasana* first, after getting up

---

47 *Hatha Yoga Pradipika* i : 64

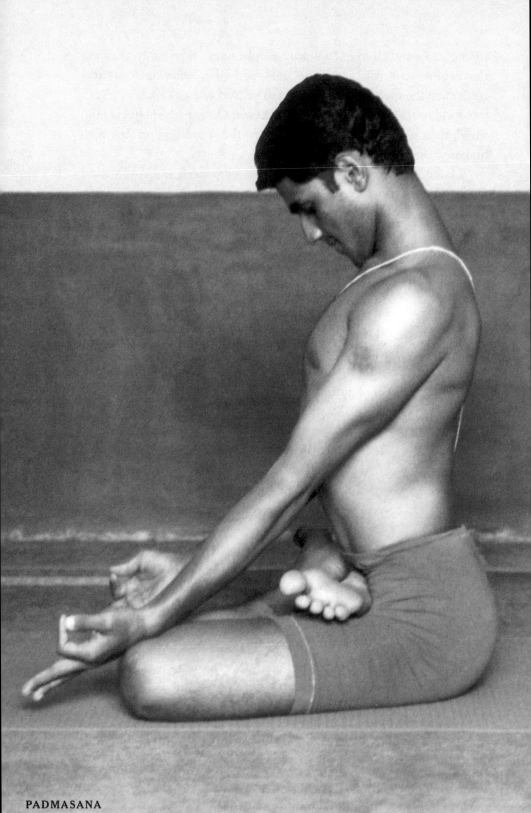

PADMASANA

before five o'clock in the morning and doing one's morning ablutions, it can lead to all sorts of trouble. This is so because ordinarily the food we eat at night, which is responsible for nourishing the body, is transformed into the seven *dhatus*. Food eaten during the day is not as effective for this purpose. In order for the food that we eat to be digested, and thereby to become one with our blood, it must join with the bile of the liver; only if the bile mixes with our food is the food digested and transformed into the seven *dhatus*. That part of what we eat that the body has no use for is eliminated in the form of feces, urine, sweat, and phlegm. For the bile produced by the liver to become one with our food, it must leave the liver. Until bile mixes with food, digests it, and then returns to its own source, namely the liver, things that lead to *pitta vikara* [activities that aggravate the liver and create excess heat] should not be engaged in. This is the rule. And this being so, if one does *Shirshasana* immediately after getting up in the morning, while the bile is still pervading the limbs of the body, and does not first do the *Surya Namaskara* and the other *asanas*, then the bile will not return to the liver, but will flow in various directions and spoil the brain. If one first practices the *Surya Namaskara* and then the other *asanas*, however, then one's blood will become hot and pure, and will flow to every part of the body, decreasing the excitement of the bile. If one then practices the seven *asanas* of *Sarvangasana*, followed by *Shirshasana*, then one's heart, intellect, and mind will evolve, preventing any harm from coming to the brain, and ensuring a long life. Hence, aspirants should never practice *Shirshasana* first. Moreover, following *Shirshasana*, they should only sit in *Padmasana* and do *pranayama* and the like, but no further *asanas*. Otherwise, danger is certain.

40. Baddha Padmasana

Baddha Padmasana is the *asana* to be practiced after *Shirshasana*. It is of two types: *Baddha Padmasana* and *Kevala* [Simple] *Padmasana*. Yoga *Mudra* occurs in *Baddha Padmasana*, and is therapeutic for diseases. *Padmasana* is useful for practices such as *dhyana* [meditation] and *pranayama*. It is also useful for the practices of the *bandhas* and *mudras*. *Baddha Padmasana* has sixteen *vinyasas*, the 8th of which is its state, and the 9th of which is Yoga *Mudra*, which is very important. Aspirants should note this.

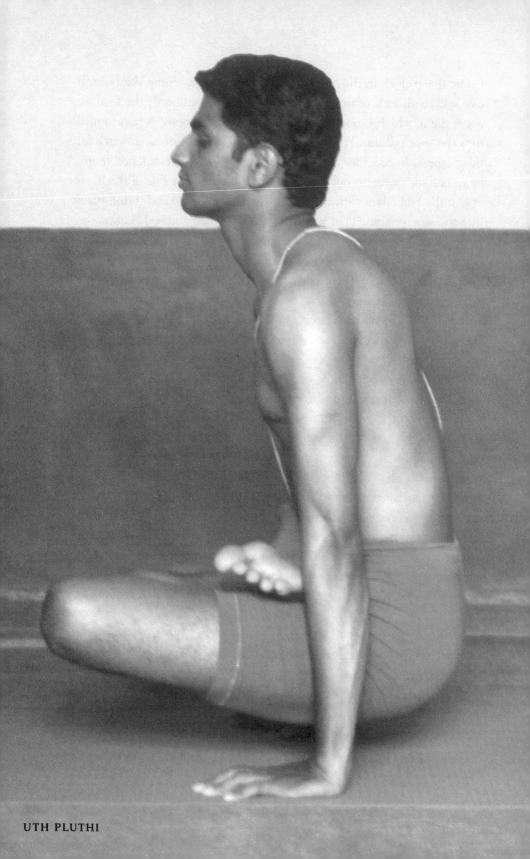

UTH PLUTHI

To begin, do the first six *vinyasas* of the first *Surya Namaskara*. Then, sit and stretch the legs out, as in *Paschimattanasana*, straighten the back and chest, and do *rechaka* and *puraka*; this is the 7th *vinyasa*. Next, place the right foot on the left thigh and the left foot on the right thigh, press the heels of both feet into the lower abdomen on either side of the navel, reach around the back, take hold of the left big toe with the left hand and the right big toe with the right hand, push the chest forward, straighten the spinal column and waist, bend the neck forward so that the chin presses into the chest, and do *rechaka* and *puraka* deeply; this is the 8th *vinyasa*. Then, doing *rechaka* slowly, place the chin on the floor, pull the navel in completely, stiffen and push the body all the way forward, and do *puraka* and *rechaka*; this is the 9th *vinyasa*, which is known as Yoga Mudra. Then, doing *puraka* and without letting go of the toes, lift the head up, sit up straight, and push the chest out; this is the 10th *vinyasa*. The next *vinyasas* follow those of preceding *asanas*.

41. PADMASANA

Kevala, or Simple, *Padmasana*, as this *asana* is also called, is useful for the practice of *pranayama, dhyana, sandhya vandana* [Brahmin ritual performed at sunrise and sunset], and *puja* [worship], among others. To practice these, one should sit in *Kevala Padmasana* after doing *Baddha Padmasana*.

METHOD

To start, follow the *vinyasas* above for *Baddha Padmasana* through the 7th *vinyasa*. Then, place the right foot on the left thigh and the left foot on the right thigh, press the heels into the lower abdomen on either side of the navel, make the knees rest on the floor, place the hands on the knees, sit up, and straighten the back, chest, and waist; this is *Padmasana*, during which *rechaka* and *puraka* should be done deeply and slowly as many times as possible. The next *vinyasas* are as those in earlier *asanas*.

BENEFITS OF BADDHA PADMASANA & PADMASANA

When in the 9th *vinyasa* of *Baddha Padmasana*, or Yoga Mudra, one should meditate upon one's chosen deity (*ishta devata*), while directing the gaze between the eyebrows and doing *rechaka* and *puraka* as much as possible. This is important. Through *Baddha Padmasana*'s practice, the liver and spleen are purified, the spinal column straightened, and the anal canal remedied. Thus, easy to do and very useful, its practice is desirable for everyone, from young to old. The greatness of *Baddha Padmasana* has been affirmed by the *Upanishads*.

The sages and seers of works such as the *Yoga Yagnavalkya* and *Yoga Vashishta* have said that the practice of *Padmasana* destroys not only diseases of the body, but great sins, as well. According to them, this is definite. Therefore, as *Padmasana* is the best and greatest of the *asanas*, and easy to practice in all respects, it should be performed by everyone.

42. UTH PLUTHI

While not an actual *asana*, *Uth Pluthi* is nevertheless highly beneficial.

METHOD

At the conclusion of *Padmasana* and without releasing the legs, press the hands firmly on the floor on either sides of the thighs and, on the force of the hands alone, lift the body up off the floor and hold, remaining in this position and doing *rechaka* and *puraka* fully as much as possible. The arms, spine, and neck should be kept completely straight, the chin tilted down a little, and the gaze should be directed on the tip of the nose. Then, jump back into the 4th *vinyasa* of the first *Surya Namaskara* and follow the *vinyasas* described in earlier *asanas*. Finally, jump through the arms, lie down, and rest for five minutes. This concludes the practice.

BENEFITS

Uth Pluthi is useful for strengthening the waist and perfecting abdominal and anal control. The three *granthis*, located in the sacrum, gradually open completely.

THE ASANAS DETAILED TO THIS POINT, WHICH ARE CURATIVE IN NATURE, HAVE now been described as completely as possible. They commonly belong to that part of the yoga method called *roga* [disease] *chikitsa*, which is useful for the cure of diseases. Of the *asanas* of the second series, which is not described in this book, some belong to *roga chikitsa* and others are *shodaka*, or purificatory. A number of the *asanas* of the third series, which also is not described here, are also purificatory, while others are capable of destroying terrible diseases, or have the power to maintain the body's firmness. The *asanas* reviewed in this book, such as *Sarvangasana*, *Halasana*, *Karnapidasana*, *Urdhva Padmasana*, *Pindasana*, *Matsyasana*, *Uttana Padasana*, *Shirshasana*, and *Padmasana*, should only be practiced after the other *asanas* have been completed. After these nine *asanas*, no further *asanas* should be done. (Those who do only a limited number of *asanas* daily should be sure to include these nine in their regimen.) If aspirants heed this advice and carefully practice the *asanas* described above, then they will have the means to prosperity, both material and spiritual.

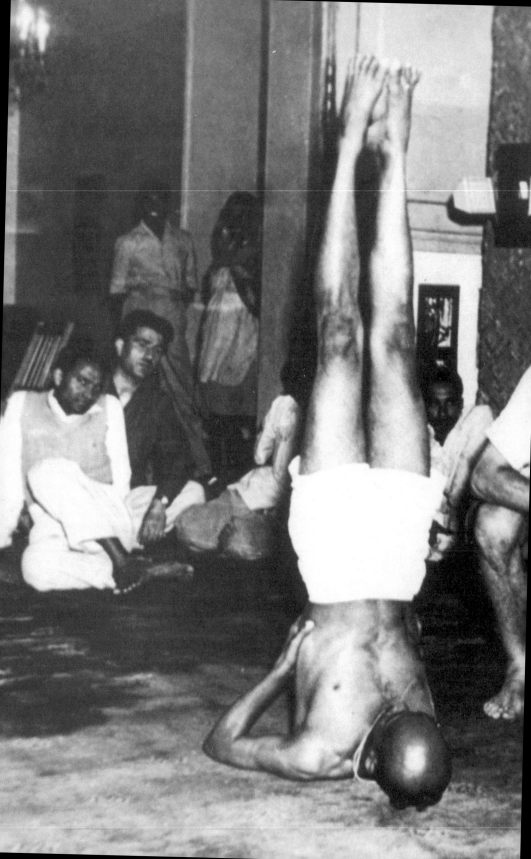

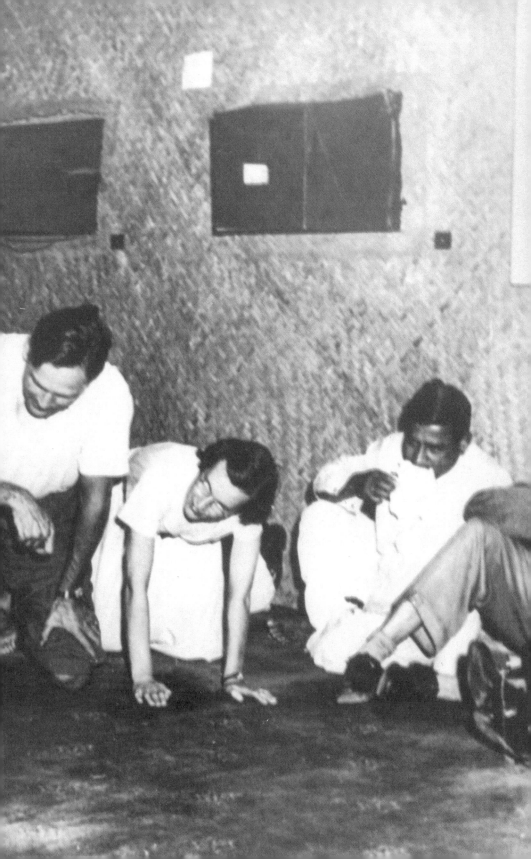

Acknowledgments

The completion of this translation of *Yoga Mala* would not have been possible without the extremely generous help of many people, in particular: Sri Vishwanath Kadam and Dr. H. L. Chandrashekar, translators; Deirdre Summerbell, editor; Swami Nityasthananda, editoral adviser; Dr. Anil Kumar, Ayurvedic adviser; Jon Hertzig, production assistant; Kathi Rota-Tebb, designer; Holton Rower, for cover and preface photographs, Stephan Crasnianski for *asana* photographs of K. Pattabhi Jois's grandson, Sharath; Vyaas Houston and the American Sanskrit Institute, Sanskrit translators; Swami Prajnatmananda and Manju Jois, for guidance; and Courtney Hayne, Kara Stern, and George Minot, proofreaders. Special thanks also to Stephanie Guest for her introduction to Jeff Seroy and Becky Saletan of North Point Press.

I am especially grateful to Sri K. Pattabhi Jois and R. Sharath for the many hours they spent working to correct the manuscript, and to Jocelyne Stern for her unending patience and support.

The efforts of this translation of *Yoga Mala* are dedicated to the lotus feet of Sri K. Pattabhi Jois, and to the loving memory of his wife, our Indian mother, Savitramma Jois.

—Eddie Stern